CONTACT YOGA®

*"Contact is a potent spiritual
medicine for your relationship."*

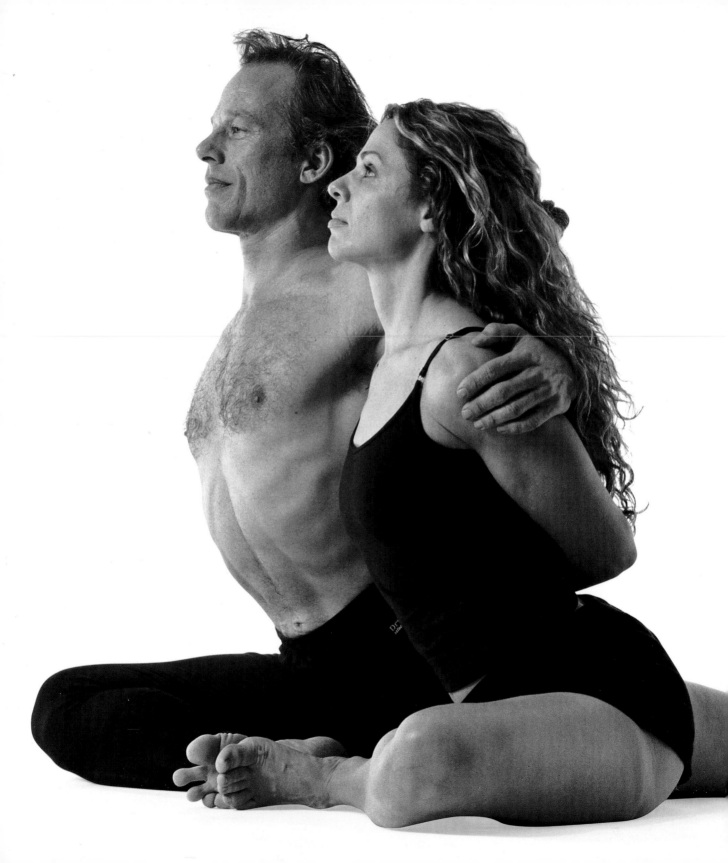

DEEPEN YOUR BOND WITH FAMILY, FRIENDS & LOVERS

CONTACT YOGA®

THE SEVEN POINTS OF CONNECTION & RELATIONSHIP

Tara Lynda Guber

WITH

Anodea Judith

PHOTOGRAPHY BY

Norman Seeff

MANDALA
PUBLISHING

San Rafael, California

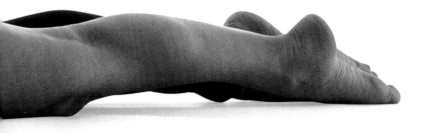

MANDALA
PUBLISHING

PO Box 3088
San Rafael, CA 94912
www.mandalaearth.com

Library of Congress Cataloging-in-Publication Data available.

ISBN: 978-1-60887-076-9

Disclaimer: Consult your doctor before beginning this yoga program, and only attempt the poses with the assistance of a trained Contact Yoga instructor. The advice presented in this book is in no way intended as a substitute for medical consultation, and the publisher disclaims any liability from, and in connection with, this program. If at any point while moving into and out of the poses described in this book you begin to feel faint, dizzy, or have physical discomfort, you should stop immediately and consult a physician.

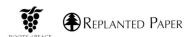

Insight Editions, in association with Roots of Peace, will plant two trees for each tree used in the manufacturing of this book. Roots of Peace is an internationally renowned humanitarian organization dedicated to eradicating land mines worldwide and converting war-torn lands into productive farms and wildlife habitats. Together, we will plant two million fruit and nut trees in Afghanistan and provide farmers there with the skills and support necessary for sustainable land use.

Manufactured in China by Insight Editions

10 9 8 7 6 5 4 3 2

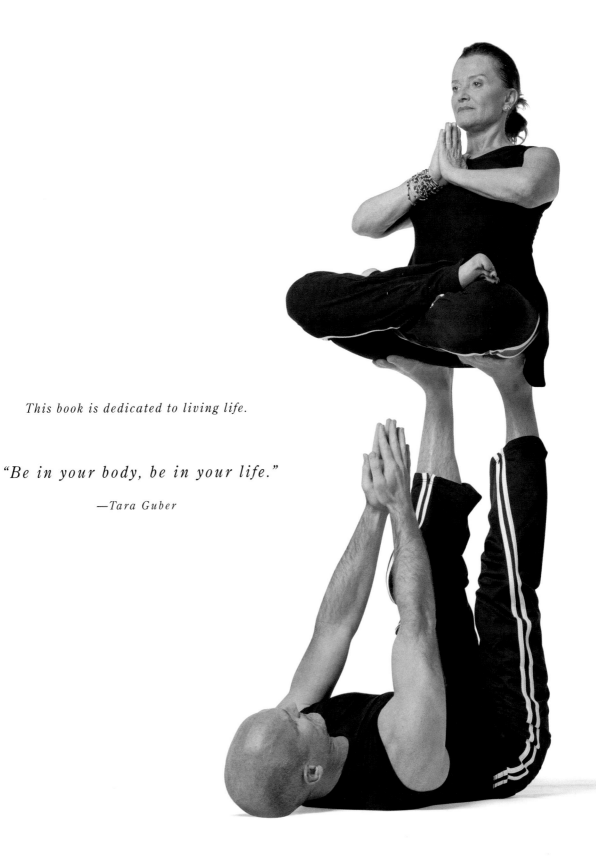

This book is dedicated to living life.

"Be in your body, be in your life."

—*Tara Guber*

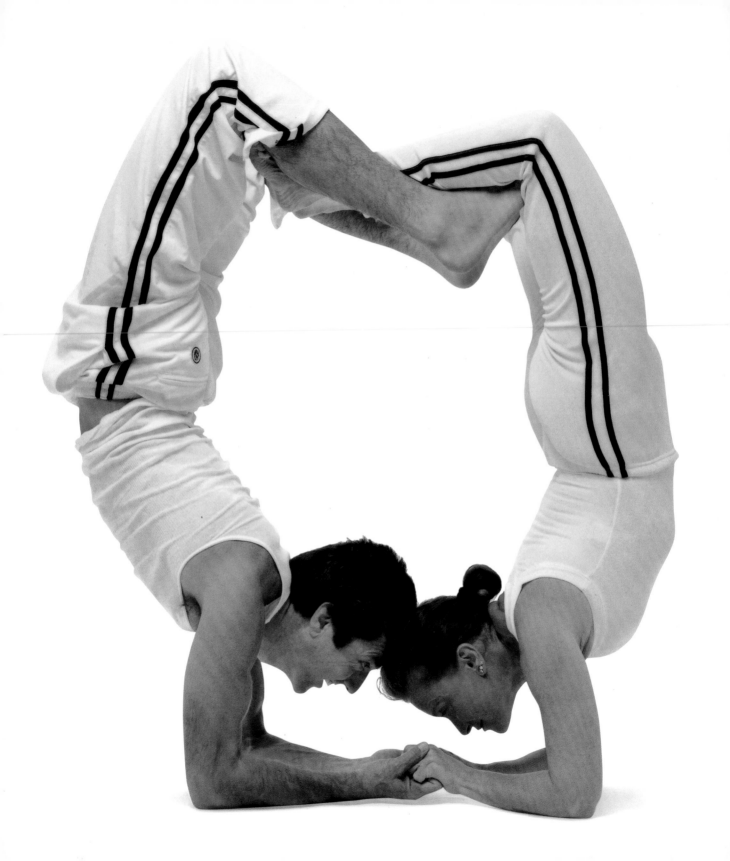

TABLE OF CONTENTS

PREFACE

We all know, at some level, that relationships are the base from which an extraordinary life of connection and happiness is built. Yet in today's modern world, life is often moving so fast that our relationships are missing the depth we crave and deserve. I believe the practices of Contact Yoga will offer you a clear path toward harnessing more of the extraordinary love, compassion, and commitment that lie within you.

Relationship is often referred to as the ultimate spiritual practice: nowhere else can you see your own beauty and challenges reflected more accurately than in the eyes of another you care for. What is the reward for all this spiritual work? An experience of greater joy and fulfillment than can ever be experienced alone! The union, connection, and intensification that relationships provide give our life meaning and purpose—whether with a child, parent, or friend, or in passionate communion with your intimate lover.

The ancient practice of yoga is defined as the union of mind, body, and spirit. What you will experience in Contact Yoga is the power of union that emerges from stepping outside of your own experience and connecting deeply with your yoga partner as you expand and transform together. When you combine the sensuality of touch with the transcendent energy available through yoga practice with your partner, you achieve ultimate communion. You literally support them as they expand their awareness through the union of mind, body, and spirit.

I have been close friends with Tara Guber for many years and am deeply touched by her passionate commitment to children through Yoga Ed., a program that brings the therapeutic and social benefits of yoga to children, teachers, and parents in public schools nationwide. Tara is a visionary yogic master who is teaching the world how to use yoga as a transformative tool for initiating deeper and more fulfilling relationships with ourselves and the world. I'm certain you'll enjoy her guidance, and I encourage you to view Contact Yoga as a compelling metaphor for the dynamics of human relationships.

Once you and a partner experience the power of Contact Yoga, your ability to be totally present, trusting, loving, and dynamic in your relationships will be transformed. Enjoy the beauty of this new path...

–Anthony Robbins

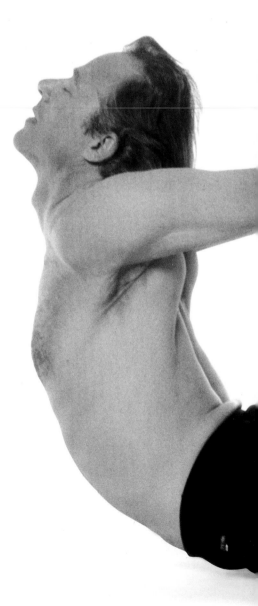

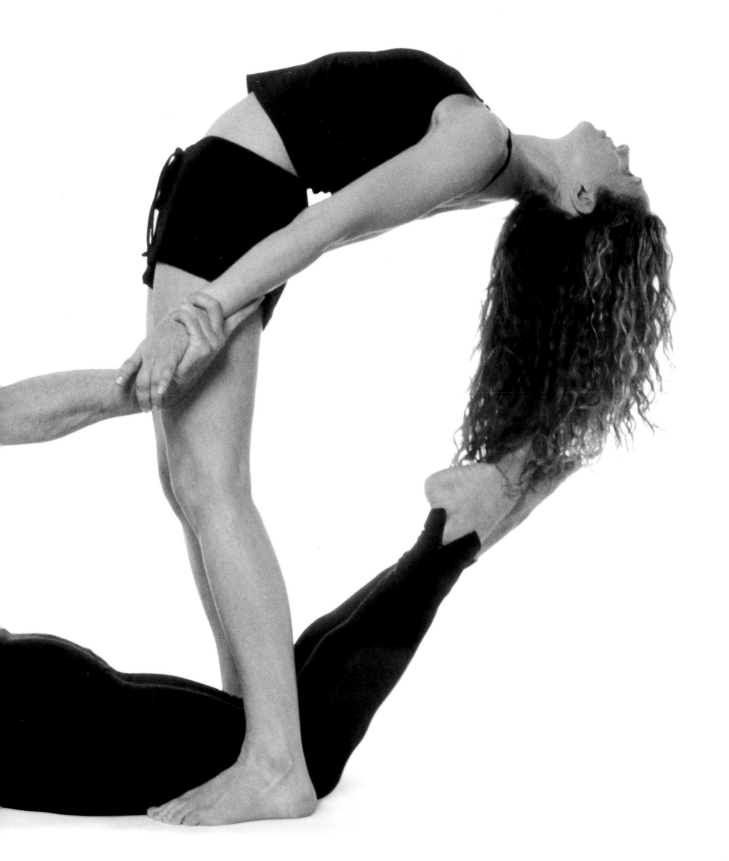

FOREWORD

The goal of all life experience and spiritual practice is union. The portal to achieving union as a state of being is dynamically engaging in the act of relationship while utilizing the full spectrum of your physical, emotional, and spiritual bodies. Once achieved, the state of union becomes the source of all true creation, illumination, revelation, and evolution: it is the universe merging with our individuated consciousness and, in so doing, the sublime context for personal transformation.

For thousands of years, yoga has been the most profound, productive, and fulfilling path to the portal of union. Within its solitary discipline, all aspects of our physically incarnated spirits are brought into alignment and harmony. Our self becomes one with the eternal "Oneness" of the universe. But as the bridge between the ancient wisdom of the East and the modern, technology-driven world of the West becomes increasingly more traveled, the gifts of yoga are finding new purpose and, I believe, are in fact evolving to a new level of energetic and spiritual expression in response to the needs of our world.

We live in shattered, fragmented times, rife with disconnection and isolation. As the tenor and cacophony of modern culture increase and intensify, we are in deep physical, emotional, and spiritual need of the healing balm of relationship. Traditional yoga provides the tools for personal oneness, but now a new form of yoga is emerging to address our modern needs by becoming the conduit for connection, activating and inspiring the relationship of one practitioner to another. This is a sacred and metaphysically catalytic act that has enormous potential to heal and transform individuals, couples, friends, and lovers. By achieving union through relationship, we become the seminal spark for a cultural evolution, empowered by spirit and in harmony with the universe.

The book you hold in your hands is a yogic portal to the profound depths of relationship. Step through and experience yoga with another, perhaps for the first time. The experience will be exhilarating, fun, challenging, cathartic, joyful, illuminating. This is a yoga that by its very nature changes you, but that change comes through and is facilitated by your "relationship" with another: you cannot access its exceptional gifts alone. You must reach out, connect, and surrender.

Contact Yoga was created in sacred service to Union by Tara Guber. What you see within these pages is her soulwork. As her friend, I have watched her on this path for many years, seeking, exploring, and, most importantly, compassionately experiencing. Contact is the journal of her pilgrimage to the frontiers of yoga and of relationship. Even if you are not a yoga practitioner, the beautifully illustrated postures of Contact Yoga are iconic and talismanic: they will speak to your unconscious and evoke within you the intimate and ecstatic nature of union between two souls that is true communion, and therefore divine. The Seven Points of Contact offer simple, practical guideposts on the path to achieving true relationship. Even off the mat, these essential qualities will serve to inform and enhance your daily life.

Sacred union is symbolized by Shiva and Shakti, the archetypical masculine and feminine of the universe, in which the singular aspects of each come together. When you become one with their dance, the exultation of spirit and the whole universe come alive in your whole being. *Contact Yoga* will show you the path of relationship, evoke this transformational spiritual ecstasy, and you will know that nothing that is born in union is impossible.

–Deepak Chopra
Author, *The Seven Spiritual Laws of Yoga*

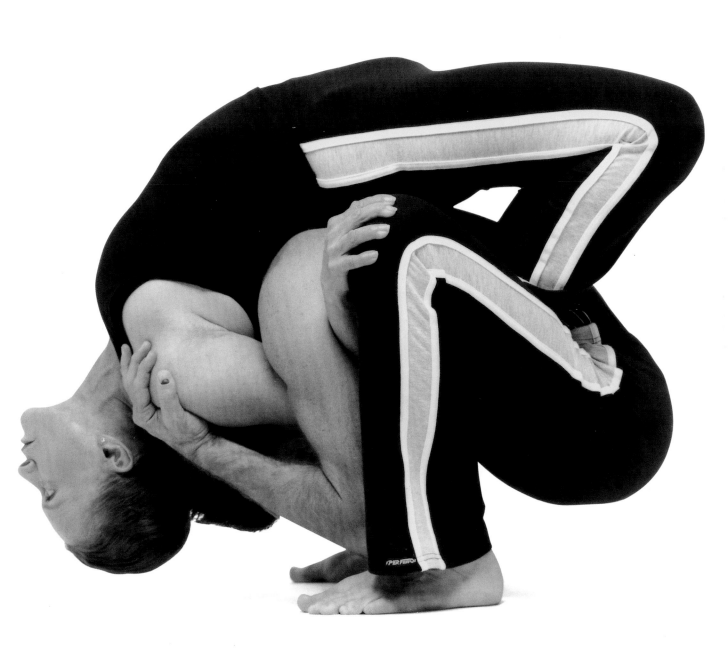

INTRODUCTION:
MY JOURNEY INTO CONTACT

I took my first yoga class more than thirty-five years ago in Norman Seeff's photography studio. At that time, I wasn't on a spiritual quest—my husband had simply injured his back. However, our yoga classes not only banished Peter's back pain but also opened a door to what would be one of the most defining, rewarding, and illuminating experiences of my life.

In those days, yoga was just beginning to catch on in the West. There were six to twelve people in the class, and we were all there to find out what yoga was really like. We explored this foreign practice with curiosity and excitement, and sought to become more flexible and fit. As we became aware of the ancient philosophy behind the practice, we began to understand our inner world and to identify the seven energy centers and systems that lay within us.

If we did this for many years, we were told, we would be well on the path to achieving enlightenment. Back then, when you admitted you practiced yoga, there were raised eyebrows and quizzical looks. But we all knew the positive changes we were feeling inside our bodies, minds, and hearts. We kept showing up for class, told our closest friends, and slowly and steadily the classes began to grow.

Today yoga is a growth industry. Its popularity has exploded in the last ten years in our increasingly health-conscious and self-involved culture. Aggressively co-opted by the fitness industry, yoga is everywhere: it now appears regularly as a vehicle to sell a host of "lifestyle" products in magazines, on television, and even on the radio. The small, open-spaced yoga class is now an endangered species. Today, there can be up to 200 people in a popular yogi's class; the mats are an inch apart and you don't know the person next to you. You don't say hello when you come in and you don't say good-bye when you leave. Many, having moved on from aerobics, are there to get the socially desirable, lean, toned "yoga body" by sweating through a demanding class. And even in this tornado of current popularity, yoga still retains the image of a solitary practice.

I don't believe that yoga is solely a fitness exercise or a practice that you do only on the mat. For me, yoga is a way of life. Yoga consciousness is reflected in everything I do each day: eating, sleeping, thinking, working, playing, and loving.

Yoga helps me reduce stress; develop a calm, quiet mind and a fit, vibrant body; increase my physical, mental, and sexual energy; improve my work performance; and deepen my relationships. Yoga is the foundation—the base of operations, if you will—of my daily routine.

During the course of my own spiritual journey, yoga has been my constant and loving companion, integrating my physical, mental, and spiritual aspects and balancing the male and female natures we all share. The practice of yoga is a potent means to understanding the greater philosophy and spiritual belief system in which it resides. Yoga has become far more than the execution of postures for me. It illuminates my personal life and, most importantly, my relationships with others.

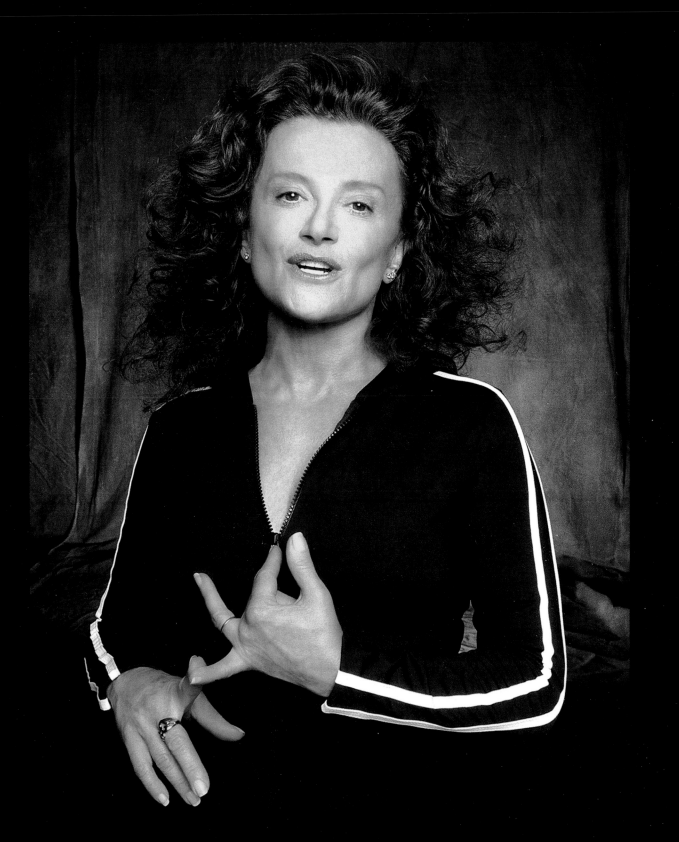

Yoga is the path that connects us with our roots and our personal history. It embraces our duality and ignites our inner fire. It catalyzes choice and interaction with others and with ourselves. It opens our hearts to unconditional love and compassion. It frees our self-expression and creativity. It reveals our insight and imagination. It lifts our true self to transcendent bliss and ecstasy.

Contact Yoga grew from my yearning to expand my practice off the mat and share the dynamics I felt in my personal practice with a partner. Even though the benefits of working with a yoga partner are well-known, I sensed that there was something beyond partner practice, something beyond the enhanced physical stretch: a heightened, more potentially transcendent and sacred experience that is centered in the heart rather than the body. I trusted this voice inside of me, followed my intuition, and began an amazing inner journey that is still going on today.

My evolution to Contact began seventeen years ago with an accomplished yogi named Tesh. We went on retreats because I wanted to both strengthen my body and deepen my practice. As a dancer and trained gymnast, Tesh was strong, flexible, and well coordinated. His yoga at the time was very interactive, with lots of partner work. When we began working together, I loved the challenge and surrender of the work, and together we really pushed the boundaries of our yoga. But he was still working me out. I said to him, "Let me do that to you."

As we practiced yoga together, I began to see that something different happened when two people connected their minds, hearts, and spirits into a posture. A heightened consciousness emerged around my movements and intention. We were moving in and out of postures without words. As soon as I became conscious of that difference, I realized how much more fun I was having because we were both doing it together. I had a companion, someone with whom I was sharing the experience, someone who could challenge me to go beyond my limits, and who could be challenged by me in turn. I had a partner who was consciously inside of the practice with me. The walls of separation between us fell away, and we laughed with the overwhelming joy of our practice. Together we created a third energy: "us," the relationship.

It is important to note here that Contact Yoga was born out of my inner intention and not my outward yoga practice. As you will see in this book, Contact goes beyond partner yoga to express and embody the deeper and more transcendent aspects of relationship. In Contact, two people's energies move into their postures to serve their desires for a deeper awareness of self and the experience of spiritual union with the self and then with another.

I believe that ultimately all we really want is a relationship. It's often our biggest challenge. We feel nervous, intoxicated, exposed, vulnerable, controlling, released, exhilarated. Contact creates a safe place to experience all of the emotions and polarities of relationships—the joys and anxieties, balance and chaos, intimacy and individuality, solitude and union. In my years of exploration and discovery within this practice, I have found Contact to be a powerful metaphor and invaluable tool in experiencing the dynamics of relationships.

Contact teaches us to ask for what we want. It requires that we communicate our hopes and desires as well as our concerns, anxieties, and even fears: I'm nervous. I feel like I'm going to fall. I'm out of balance. Are you there? Are you holding me? Contact breaks down the barriers of physical connection, opens the door to emotional connection, clears the channels of energetic connection, and merges you with the transcendent spirit. I like to say that the essence of Contact is constant awareness of your partner. In the process of moving through the postures, one can actually overcome fear, form trust, increase communication, and deepen intimacy. As you embrace the full potential of each Contact posture, you will experience a sublime expression of transcendent union.

Practicing yoga and meditation does not guarantee a great relationship. I believe it comes down to willingness and intention. Are you willing to be vulnerable and open? Are you willing to move beyond your boundaries? And when you do so, what is your intention?

As I sought to understand the benefits of Contact and the powerful and transformational flows of energy it triggered, I saw an association between relationships and the seven energy centers of the body called chakras. The more I studied, the more evident the parallels became. Relationships follow the same energy system as the chakras, moving from a place of foundation and trust to one of surrender and freedom. After much exploration and refining, I was able to define the Seven Points of Contact, a system that expresses the connection between the chakras and relationship. In forthcoming chapters, we will explore the Seven Points of Contact in depth.

–Tara Lynda Guber

"Be impeccable with your word.
Don't take anything personally.
Don't make assumptions.
Always do your best."

—*Don Miguel Ruiz from* The Four Agreements

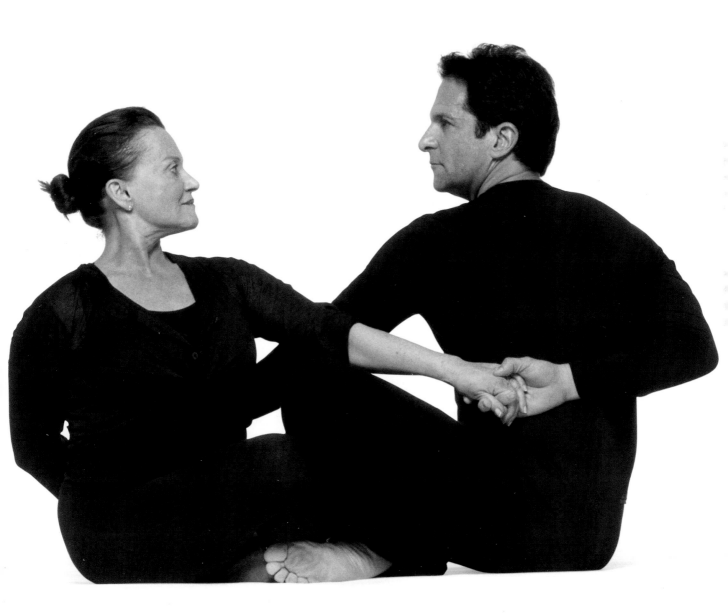

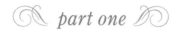

part one

CONTACT

BACKGROUND & GUIDELINES

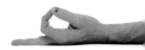

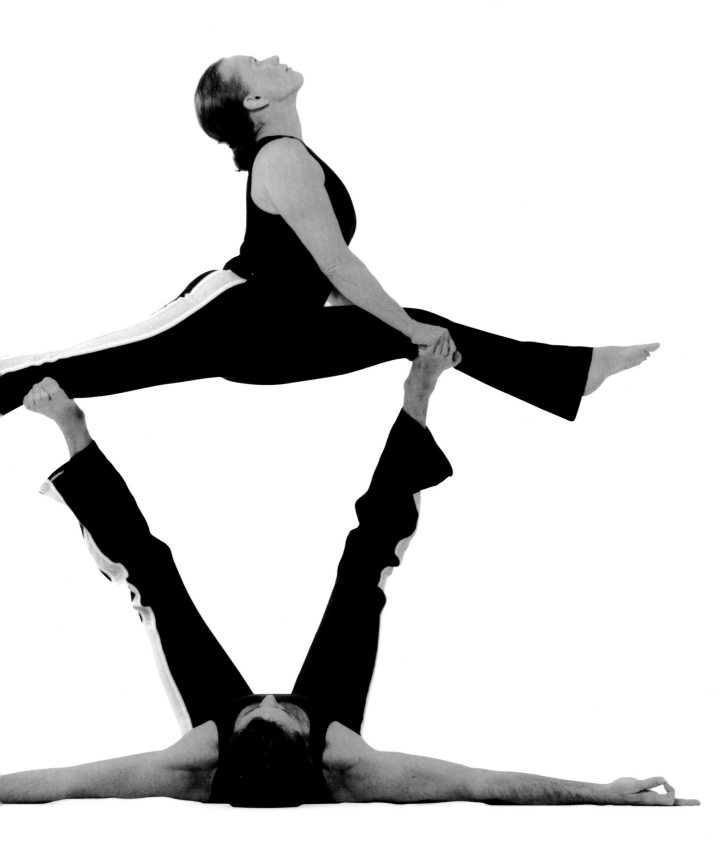

CHAPTER 1

THE SEVEN POINTS OF
CONTACT

⑦ UNION: Surrender, Service, Freedom

⑥ VISION: Intuition, Focus, Creativity

⑤ COMMUNICATION: Conversation, Connection, Honesty

④ LOVE: Forgiveness, Compassion, Acceptance

③ COMMITMENT: Will, Discipline, Responsibility

② PASSION: Sensuality, Pleasure, Desire

① TRUST: Foundation, Integrity, Security

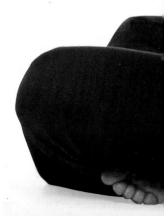

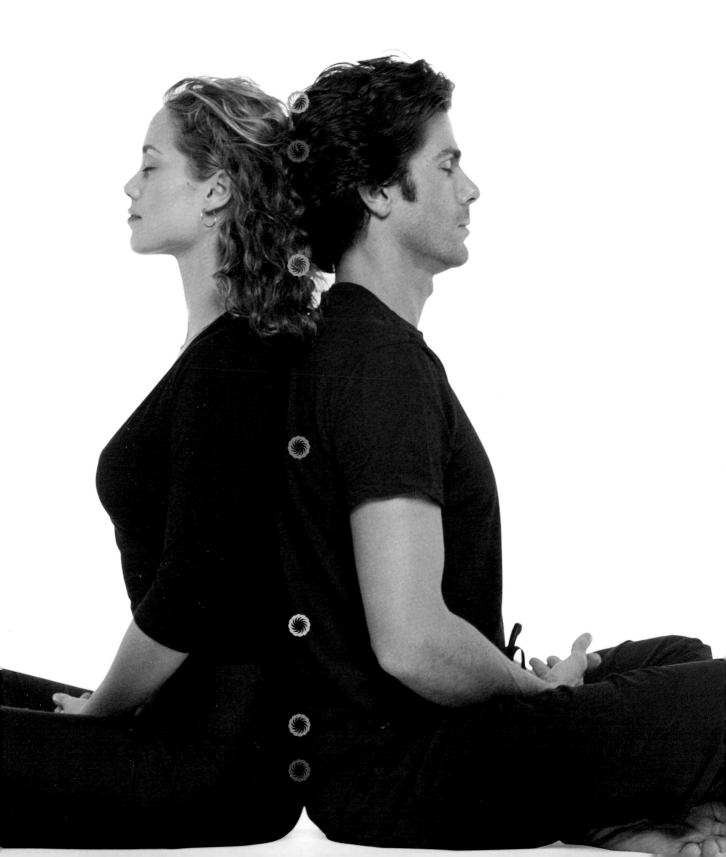

*"The privilege of a lifetime
is being who you are."*

—*Joseph Campbell*

When I brought my understanding of these Seven Points into both my yoga practice and my relationships, I found the impact to be profound. I now had a more insightful and spiritual way to think and feel about the joys and challenges of relationships. I developed a new vocabulary, which I call the language of Contact, for use in my practice and in my life. This understanding and language were grounded in and expressed through the postures of Contact Yoga. Contact gave me a way to experience and channel these powerful energies and focus them on evolving and transforming my relationships, first with myself and my Contact partner, and then with everyone in my life.

I have found that certain Contact poses evoke the particular qualities of each of the Seven Points. By practicing these postures with shared intention and dedication, you and your partner can enhance and build the specific energy of a Point in you, your partner, and your relationship.

The postures of Contact Yoga are the embodiment of two separate identities and souls joining to create something that neither could create alone: the Two who become One. To achieve this sacred union, trust, surrender, and service must replace fear, power, and control. Each partner must do his or her own inner work in preparation for cooperative work.

Our acceptance of and commitment to doing our own inner work are essential and necessary components to realizing a fulfilling Contact experience. Your dedication to your own personal growth is to be felt and honored by your partner, in turn inspiring him or her to do the same. Until we achieve harmony and wholeness within ourselves and develop trust and communication with our partners, our experience of relationships both on and off the mat will be limited and unfulfilling.

In this book, we will explore how the philosophy, practices, and meditations of Contact Yoga can empower you in your quest for an enlightened relationship.

In addition to clear, illustrated instructions, you will see and read about the direct experience of practitioners of Contact Yoga.

Most importantly, I want to inspire and support you in the belief that you can evolve and transform your relationship by taking responsibility for your own intentions and actions, sharing them openly and compassionately with your partner, and being receptive when your partner does the same.

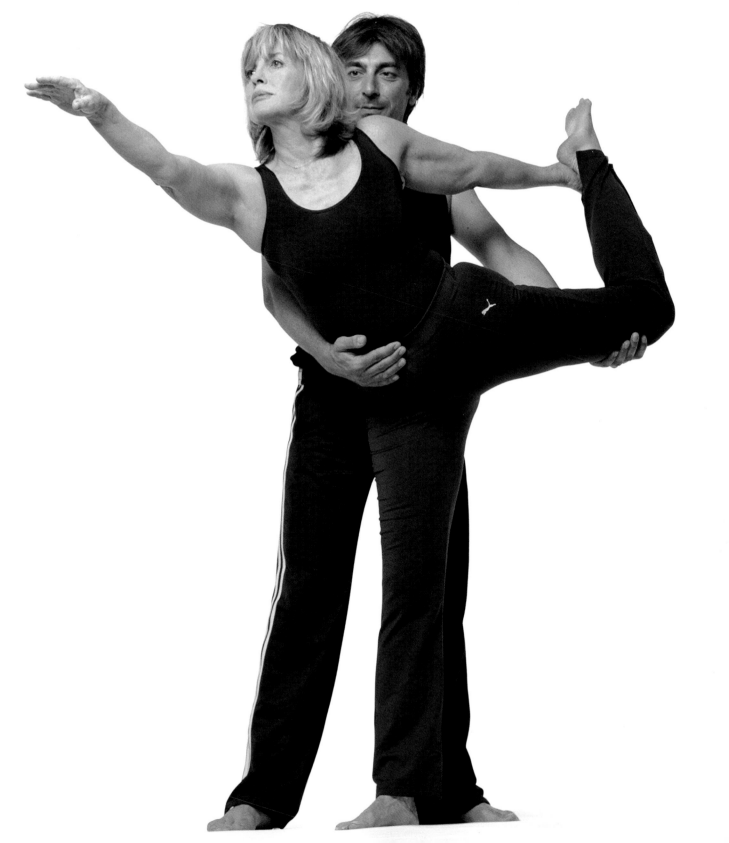

HOW TO USE THIS BOOK

THIS IS A DIFFERENT KIND OF YOGA BOOK

Unlike other forms of yoga practice, the objective in Contact Yoga is not to mirror the perfect form of an ancient discipline, nor is it the serious-minded quest for absolute perfection in the postures. In fact, it's quite the opposite. It's about crossing barriers and boundaries, bold exploration, trial and error, exciting creativity, spontaneity, and invention. But more than anything else, Contact Yoga is about fun.

This book is designed to be both instructional and inspirational. In each section you will find a beginning-level posture with detailed instructions that anyone can follow and benefit from. Some postures may look difficult but are actually easy to achieve. Others are more advanced and are best tried by yogis with some years of experience. I include these not only because they are compelling examples of the dynamic beauty of Contact, but also to inspire you, to show you what can be accomplished with patience, practice, and discipline. Just like relationships, no two Contact Yoga practices are alike. For me, that's what makes it so special.

I encourage you to start with the basics. Then, once you and your partner are comfortable, try things; explore, play, see what works for you. I guarantee that you will surprise yourself.

There is another aspect that sets Contact Yoga apart from other practices. Often in modern yoga practice, there is considerable emphasis on outward form and the physical benefits—high flexibility, sweating, and "perfection"—but not on expressing and sharing the inner experience of yoga. In relationships, our inner dialogue can be so revealing of our true emotional and spiritual state. It is the same with Contact. Your communication with your partner is not only about what you are doing but also what you are feeling, and is an absolutely essential part of the practice. In this book, yogi practitioners of all ages and from all levels appear in Contact poses and speak about their personal experiences. Use these conversations as examples of what can be achieved in Contact, or as a launching place for your own dialogues. Remember this: the more you express your feelings and communicate them to your partner with love, compassion, and truth, the more your Contact Yoga practice (and your relationship) will grow and evolve.

"It is our duty, as men and women, to proceed as though the limits of our abilities do not exist."

—*Pierre Teilhard de Chardin*

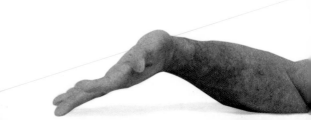

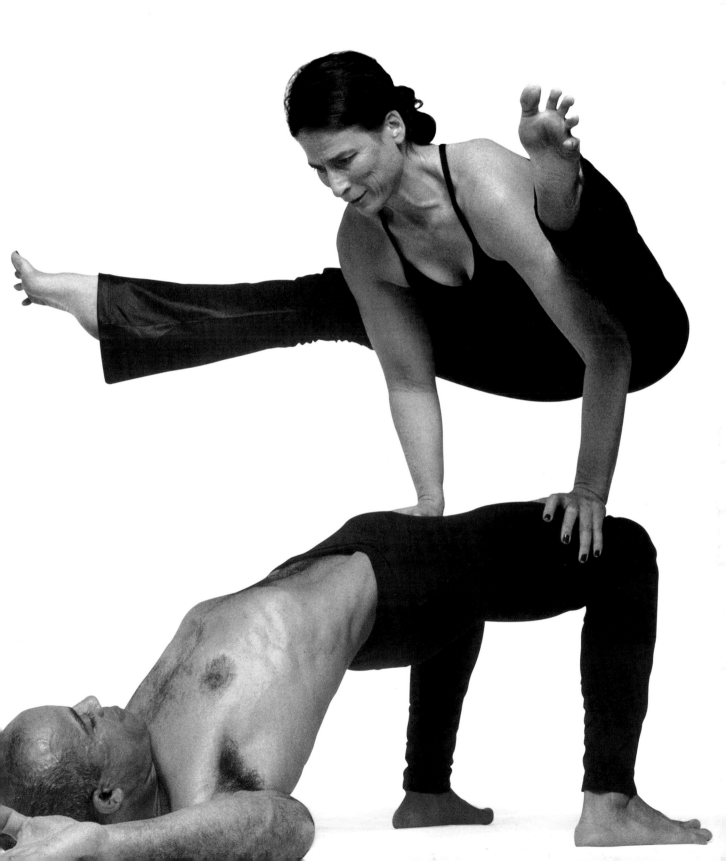

CHAPTER 2

POINTS, POSTURES &
PRACTICE

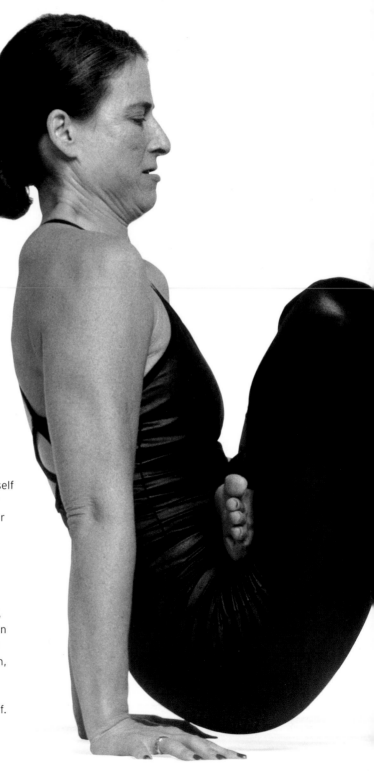

Relationship, for those who truly practice it, is a potent form of yoga. Its parallels to yoga's spiritual practice are many: it stretches you to greater flexibility, furthers your personal awakening, and leads you to your highest self. It requires dedication, discipline, and daily practice. Its goal, like the true meaning of the Sanskrit word *yoga*, is union. In fact, Contact Yoga is a kind of foreplay for union, a means of dissolving the false separation between self and other, and through that path, experiencing unity with all that is.

Traditional yoga is a series of practices for aligning yourself with core spiritual principles. It hones body and mind to their highest potential. Whether practicing postures, directing your breath, or stilling your mind in meditation, yoga is largely a solitary practice. You may work one-on-one with a teacher, go to a class, or practice with others, but yoga is a system primarily designed for individuals to grapple with their own path to enlightenment.

Partner yoga, a fairly recent movement in the yoga world, utilizes postures that two people do simultaneously, and often symmetrically. In partner yoga, two people might play with balance, weight, twisting, lifting, or pushing, but most often, they are doing the same pose at the same time. The focus is usually on the pose itself, rather than what's happening between the partners. Contact Yoga is about relationship itself.

Contact enhances the awareness with which you see, understand, and relate to another person. To practice

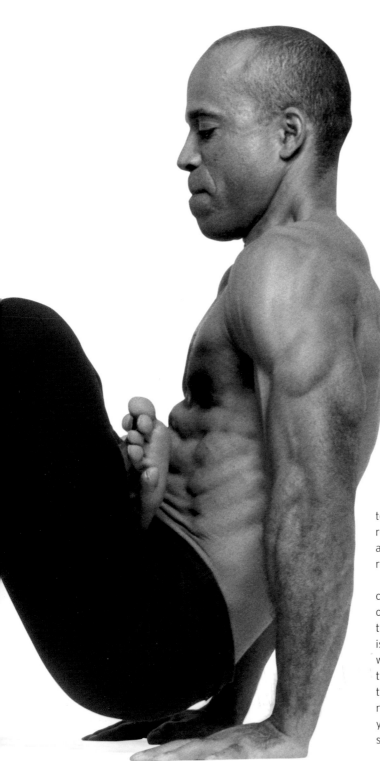

Contact is to experience yoga, lovemaking, and chiropractic and mutual massage all at once. This kind of connection is not subtle, wishy-washy, or abstract. It is intense, focused, and wildly therapeutic.

Contact Yoga explores that mysterious edge where two people connect physically, emotionally, and spiritually. Contact breaks down the barriers that keep us separated. Two people practicing Contact, whether they're just friends, passionate lovers, yogis and yoginis in a class together, or long-term life partners, discover their inherent patterns of relating. No matter how long a couple has been together, an hour of Contact is bound to open new frontiers in their relationship.

While there are many spiritual practices that two people can do at the same time, such as meditation, yoga, chanting, or even gardening, there are far too few spiritual practices that focus on enhancing a relationship itself. Contact Yoga is a spiritual practice for learning how to relate to another with balance, power, and clarity. It teaches you to dissolve the boundaries that create separation while still remaining true to yourself—certainly the most basic challenge of any relationship. This miraculous practice transforms your body, your psyche, and your relationships, a critical evolutionary step in the practice of yoga and the art of awakening.

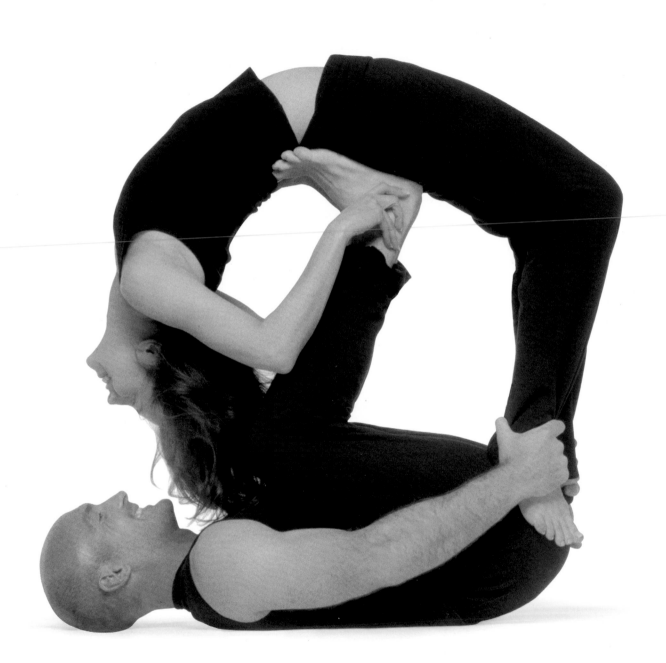

THE SEVEN POINTS OF
CONTACT

C an you trust that your partner will hold steady while you expand? Can you commit to giving support so your partner can fly? Can you communicate your fears and needs when your world is turned upside down? Do you see eye to eye? Do you have fun together, laughing and releasing, finding pleasure and passion?

These questions arise in Contact, and, sooner or later, in any relationship. They reflect basic issues important to us all: trust, passion, commitment, love, communication, vision, and union. These emotions correspond to the chakras in yoga, which are aligned along the spine.

Chakras are seven vortices of energy swirling along the spine from root to crown. They act as gateways between the inner and outer worlds. They are the seven windows to the soul, from where the light of consciousness shines out. They are also the organizational centers that manage and transform the energies all around us to be used by the soul. An ancient map for the journey of awakening, the chakra system is the spiritual blueprint for the human nervous system. To make contact with these centers is to open the gates to your inner temple, the very temple that you share with your partner.

The chakra system is a metaphor for the workings of the inner world. When you look at the way chakras affect relationships and combine the map of the chakra system with the practice of Contact Yoga, you have an elegant set of principles that we call the Seven Points of Contact. These are places of connection where important energies flow back and forth between people. The Seven Points of Contact describe the essential bonds that make a relationship vital, healthy, and complete. If any of these Points are missing, the relationship suffers. When each Point is open and connected, the relationship thrives.

These Seven Points form the foundation of Contact Yoga.

Where do you really connect in your relationship? Where do you fail to make contact? Where do you want improvement? Perhaps you are strongly passionate but fail in your communication. Or perhaps the passion is missing, even though your commitment is still strong. Maybe you find it hard to trust, yet long for a deeper union. These are the issues common to most relationships, issues that emerge in the practice of Contact Yoga.

Trust, Passion, Commitment, Love, Communication, Vision, and Union—these are the things we long for, these are the treasures of relationship. We know their gifts well, yet each has its challenges—hidden places of conflict that interfere with a solid connection. We must acknowledge these shadow aspects if we are to transform them. The Swiss psychologist Carl Jung once said, "We don't become enlightened by chasing after figures of light, but by making the darkness conscious." By bringing our shadow elements to light, we remove the barriers that keep us from union.

The shadow aspects of the Seven Points of Contact represent the places where we hold back, our fears, confusions, insecurities, and struggles. They are places not to be avoided, but embraced and transformed into avenues for greater contact. Then we can harvest their gifts—the precious pearls that so powerfully enhance relationship. When passion and desire arise, it can be frightening, but if we surrender to the flow of energy, we experience the joy that passion and pleasure bring. To risk vulnerability is to find intimacy. To have clear communication, we must risk honesty, but when we do, the reward is inspiration and deeper rapport. To see someone clearly, we need to pierce through the illusions of projections and assumptions and receive the gift of clarity.

THE SEVEN POINTS
WITH THEIR ASSOCIATED GIFTS AND CHALLENGES

point of contact	*challenge*	*gift*
① TRUST	Fear	Safety
② PASSION	Surrender	Joy
③ COMMITMENT	Struggle	Freedom
④ LOVE	Vulnerability	Intimacy
⑤ COMMUNICATION	Distance	Rapport
⑥ VISION	Illusion	Clarity
⑦ UNION	Ego	Grace

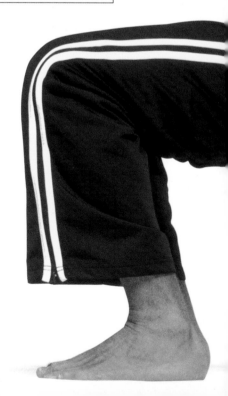

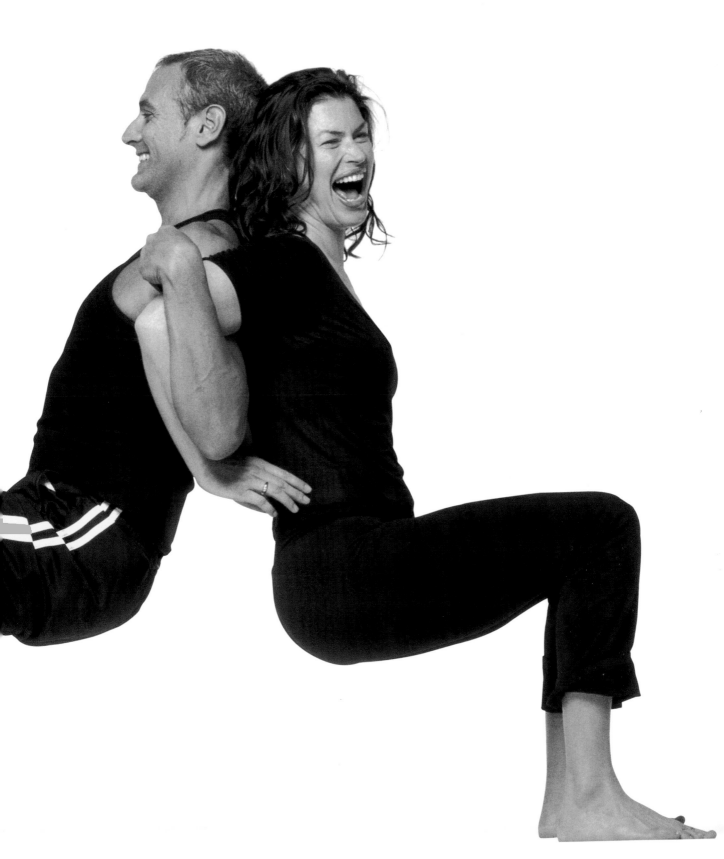

CHAPTER 3

POINTS IN
PRACTICE

The Seven Points of Contact have a natural order, building energy through the chakras, from base to crown. In working these Points and developing your practice and experience, begin with the first Point and work your way through the system. This channels the *prana*, or energy, in logical fashion, toward the goal of union.

It's easy to see what happens when these Points are skipped over, or not consciously created in the building of relationship. Without trust, passion can lead you to betrayal; without passion, commitment is an obligation; without commitment, love doesn't have the protection it needs to deepen; without love, communication can be hurtful; without communication, there is no shared vision; and without all of these, union is incomplete.

Yet each Point is always active within each of the other Points. Communication, for example, is necessary for trust to form, for love to deepen, and for commitments to be clarified. Love enhances passion and invites trust. Vision supports commitment and unites partners in a common goal. And the more you transcend your ego and allow yourself to flow into union, the more each of these Points will be enhanced in turn.

When the attitude of each Point is embraced fully in the postures, the chakras align—both within yourself and between you and your partner. The vital energy, or *kundalini*, then rushes up the spine, expanding your experience together as each of the chakras opens and releases. Old patterns of limiting beliefs and feelings of isolation diminish. The mind surrenders, the body expands, and the spirit soars.

It's important to keep the principles of Contact in mind as you practice, for it's not just the poses, but the intention within the poses that allows two people to experience the true magic of this work. If you really work the Seven Points as you practice, you will find that Contact is a potent spiritual medicine for your relationship.

Each of the following chapters presents a description of the principles of each Point, as well as its associated postures and the practice. The practice gives you simple exercises that can be carried into the postures themselves. Avoid rushing into the postures without first establishing the Points of Contact in each chapter. Think of the postures as playground equipment—something to climb upon. The gifts you harvest from the practice are the direct result of your attitude. The more you can focus your intention on the principle in question, the greater your rewards will be—for you, your partner, and your relationship.

Relationship is not performance art and neither is Contact Yoga, even though the poses can be quite beautiful. Let go of preconceived notions about performing—doing the poses perfectly or being the perfect partner. Don't worry if you aren't flexible enough, strong enough, or do not have a perfect body. These postures are more about connection than perfection, more about exploration than expectation. As you work through the poses of the Seven Points of Contact, take your experience into your relationship in a spirit of openness, without judgment.

Contact Yoga unfolds in the moment. You discover things about yourself as you explore, and you will laugh at yourself as you fall. Chances are, you won't be able to hold on to your old ways of being; you won't be able to control, run, hide, or manipulate. But you will be able to go at your own pace, testing and exploring together.

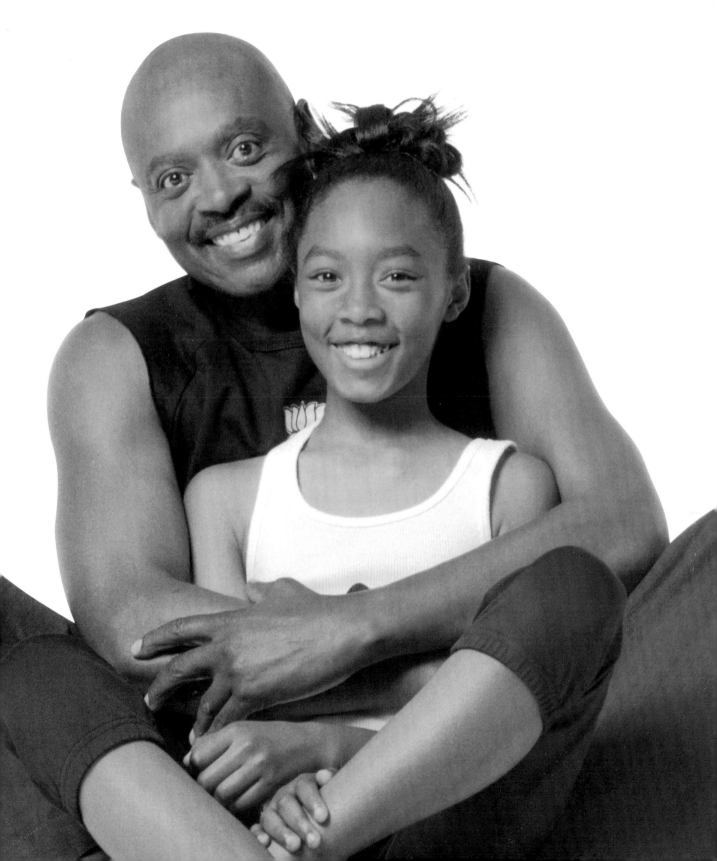

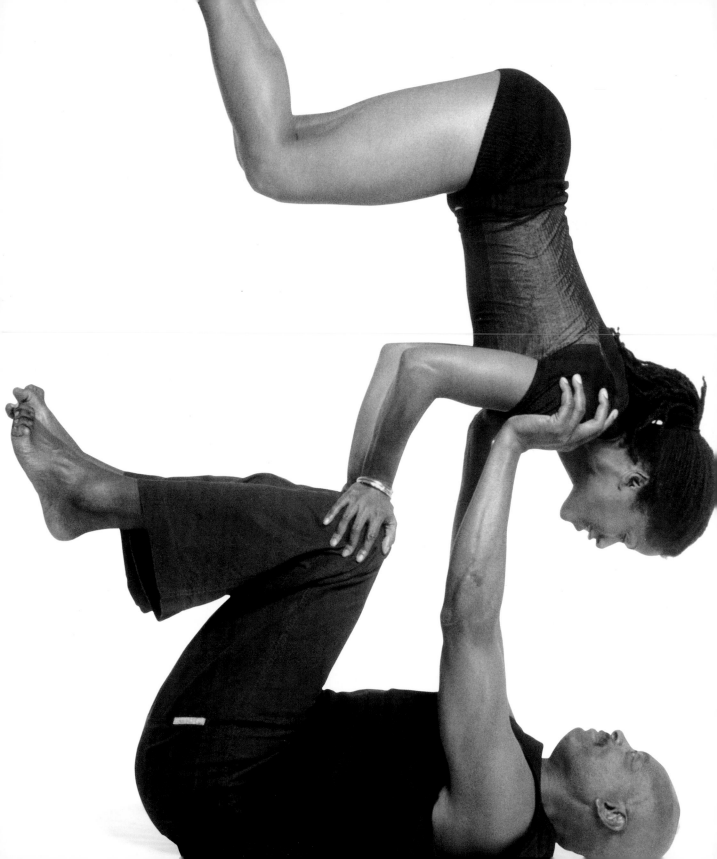

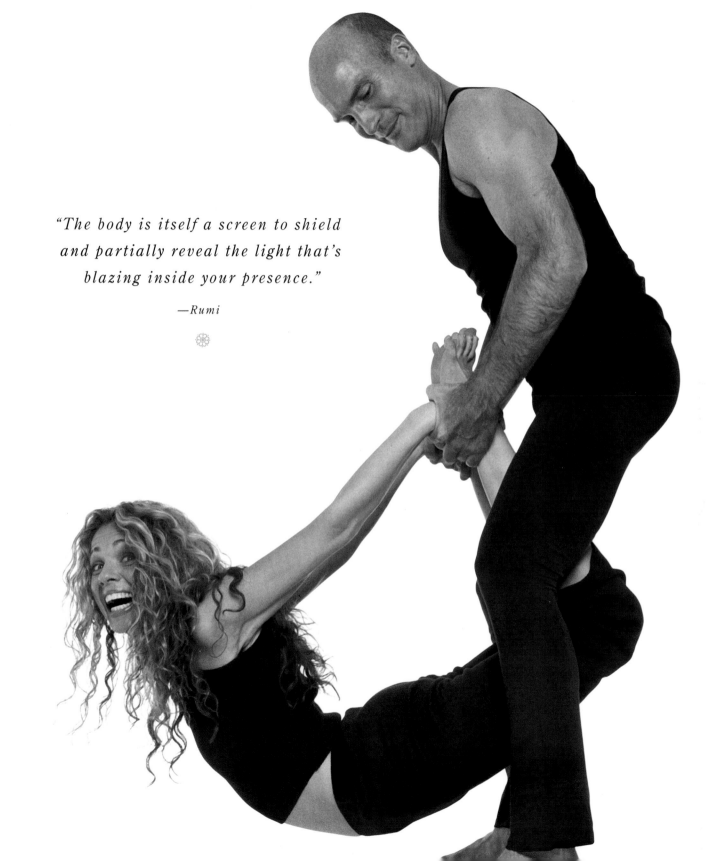

"*The body is itself a screen to shield and partially reveal the light that's blazing inside your presence.*"

—*Rumi*

CHAPTER 4

GENERAL GUIDELINES FOR
APPROACHING CONTACT

Build upon Each Step

Practice the Points of Contact one step at a time. Establish your principles of trust and make them the foundation of your practice, and let the rest unfold. As you learn each Point, apply it to whatever pose you are doing. You will see how each of them is present in the formation of any pose: all postures require trust, commitment, communication, or vision. All lead to union, create passion, or enhance love.

Begin with Yourself

Each Point of Contact with your partner begins within you. Before you can trust another, you must trust yourself. If you don't have passion for life, you won't have it for your partner. Before you can pleasure another, you must be in touch with your own pleasure. If you can't listen to your own truth, you won't have clear communication.

Share Your Own Experience

You may want to point things out to your partner about his or her behavior—just as you always do—but it is far more fruitful to share your own experience and invite your partner to share his or hers. You will be acting in the spirit of discovery; the experience will remain fun and exciting. Speak your truth, but state it from your own experience. In other words, you might say, "I can feel the place where I resist," rather than "I see you are resisting again." "I feel scared I may fall" is more inviting to your partner than "You never support me the way I want," which provokes defensiveness. Intimacy is the sharing of one's interior without judgment or blame.

Maintain Your Own Yoga Practice

A solid practice and understanding of yoga is the basic language of Contact, just as Italian is the basic language of Italy. The more fluently your body speaks the language of yoga, the deeper your Contact and the more you will find an ecstatic place to share the fruits of your personal practice.

This is not meant to exclude those new to yoga; Contact with beginners and advanced together offers a worthwhile experience for both. But the real jewels of Contact, just as in solitary yoga, are found when two bodies, honed from years of personal yoga practice, come together to combine their yoga in Contact. Beginners who do Contact quickly discover this. They want to do Contact again and again, but they are also inspired to go home and do their own practice, so they can bring greater strength and flexibility to the mat with their partner.

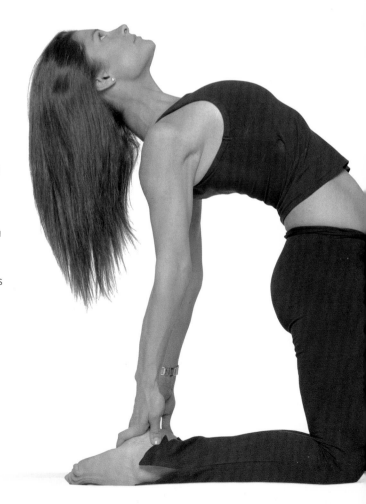

Create Sacred Space

Contact Yoga is an exquisite date with your partner. Create a space to really explore. Take time to honor each other. Be open to accepting and embracing each other's identity, right where it is. Be in the now with your partner; focus not on how it should or could be, but how it is. Surrender to the outcome; drop all expectations.

Take Responsibility

If you are working your own body, you are working your partner. If it's good for you, it's probably good for your partner. What you experience will tell you more about you than about your partner, and that's the best place to start. Check in.

Listen. Feel. You evoke in each other that which has to be uncovered. Having a good time is a very likely outcome, but make it your responsibility rather than your partner's.

Use Visualizations

Engage your intuition and imagination. Don't be bound by forms, but meet what is. Experiment. Be creative. Imagine the colors of the chakras, or the energies of two becoming one. Open your vision.

Empower the Positive

Celebrate and embody the positive aspects of the experience. Refrain from judging, criticizing, complaining, or focusing on the negative. Focus on what you want, not what you don't want. What you focus on, you invite.

Get Out of Your Head and Into Your Heart

Contact is not a competition. It is a gutsy practice of intimate risk, physical challenge, and spiritual awakening. It is an experience, not a concept. Leave your head at home, and come into the present moment of the body's energetic and sensate experience. As Fritz Perls, the cofounder of Gestalt therapy, used to say, "Lose your mind and come to your senses."

Work Your Edge

Contact happens in the ever-narrowing space between yourself and another. It takes you to your edge; it takes your partner to his or her edge. This vital, uncharted frontier is the gateway to the mystery of relationship. Learn to hang out on that edge, communicate from the precipice, and meet your partner there. It may not be comfortable, but it will be expanding.

Have Fun!

Use the postures like a playground and be kids again, without preconceived notions about how it's supposed to go. Return to the innocence of a beginner's mind. Laugh, play, and explore.

CHAPTER 5

CREATING A SACRED SPACE

In preparing for your Contact practice, it is important to set aside time to come together in a quiet, uncluttered space. Remember to first feed the dog or cat, make sure your children are taken care of, turn off the phones, and get everything out of the way that might distract you. Put on your favorite CD or light some candles to set the mood.

Make a list of things you would like to bring into your yoga space. These may include: incense, candles, music, flowers, a yoga mat or carpet, yoga straps, a blanket, water, a towel, and a hair band.

To begin openly communicating and connecting, you may read a favorite poem, share what your day was like, or dance to your favorite music. It is fun to surprise your partner with something new or unlike you; don't be afraid to show your wild side. Be conscious of the words you use when communicating with your partner; words have impact, so use them wisely. You will soon get to a place in your practice where words are not necessary. The flow of energy and trust alone will move you from one posture to the next.

"Out beyond ideas of right doing and wrong doing, there is a field. I'll meet you there."

—*Rumi*

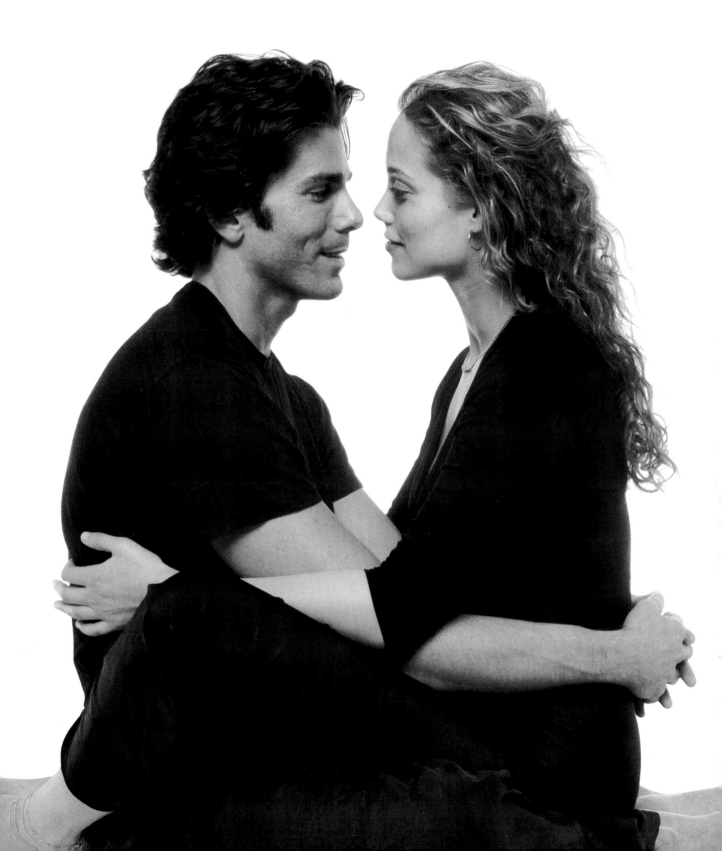

A CONTACT PARTNER
MEDITATION

Begin by sitting cross-legged, back-to-back with your partner. Align your spines from root to crown, feeling the places where your backs make contact as well as the places where they are not touching. Try to make as much contact as possible, not only along the spine but across your shoulders, midback, buttocks, neck, and head. Rest your hands on your knees or clasp them in front of you and begin to breathe. Drop your shoulders, relax your chest, and connect calmly with your partner.

As you reach each Point, feel it in your body; explore what it means to you. For example:

- *Do you trust yourself? Do you trust others?*
- *Remember a time when you really trusted someone. Visualize that moment and remember that feeling. Let it fill you completely.*
- *From the radiance of that feeling, begin to open to trust in all aspects of your life.*
- *Feel how you can better trust yourself, trust others, and trust the universe.*
- *Breathe into the ball of red light and connect through your spine to your partner's as you sit surrounded and immersed in the energy of trust.*
- *In the same manner, move through all of the Seven Points according to the guidance written here:*

First Point: TRUST

Place your attention at the first Point of Contact, at the base of the spine. Imagine two red, glowing balls of energy, emanating from each of your spines, flowing into one another. Each sphere remains distinct, yet they make contact with each other, blending their edges into one.

This Point relates to trust. Imagine that your body is solid enough to provide support for your partner, and that your partner can provide support for you. What does it feel like in your body when you know you can trust your partner? What does it feel like when you know you can trust yourself? Allow this trust to form a foundation for your practice and your relationship. Enjoy the feeling of being held by that trust.

Second Point: PASSION

Next, place your attention on the sacral area of the spine. Press your sacrum against the back of your partner's sacrum. Feel how you have to flex and wiggle your spine to make contact here. Let that movement be light and playful, bringing pleasure and ease. Take a breath and smile. Reach through your senses and really feel your partner. Visualize a glowing sphere of orange light moving toward a similar sphere in your partner, each flowing into the other.

This is the second Point of Contact, which relates to passion. Where do you feel passionate about life? Where do you feel passion in your relationship? How do you experience that in your body?

Breathe into your Point of Contact and connect with your passion and desire. Imagine them as a river of feeling flowing into a stream of excitement between you and your partner. Pay special attention to all the sensations in your body, allowing the energy of passion to flow through your entire being.

Third Point: COMMITMENT

Next, bring your attention up to your solar plexus, center of power and will. Imagine a glowing, yellow fire emanating from this point, radiating in all directions. Use your will to press this part of your back into your partner's back and imagine the sparks and flames from each of your fires intertwining.

This Point relates to commitment. Make a commitment to being fully present, focused, and attentive to your practice with your partner. Feel how your intention focuses your energy and allows you to really be there for him or her. Where does your body hold back from that commitment? Where do you feel struggle within? Use your will to focus your energy into this point, feeling how your commitment can free the flow of energy to be single-pointed and powerful.

Fourth Point: LOVE

Next, focus your attention on the area of your chest and heart. Take a moment to listen to your heartbeat. Take a deep breath and listen to the air flowing in and out as you breathe. Coordinate your breathing with your partner's breath, inhaling and exhaling together. Feel your backs expand and contract with each breath.

This Point of Contact is related to love itself. Relax your shoulders and soften the area around your heart. Imagine the energy of the heart expanding with love, a green, glowing sphere of love widening with each breath. Feel it expand until it can encompass your whole body and then expand it to encompass the body of your partner. See this field of love surrounding you both.

Open your heart to the softness of caring and intimacy, with full acceptance of yourself just as you are. Extend that acceptance and caring to your partner. Allow compassion and forgiveness to flow from your heart, softening your chest with each breath. Imagine that each movement in your practice is guided by a feeling of love, radiating from your heart. This love asks nothing in return, but simply emanates from a spirit of openness and compassion, intimacy and acceptance.

Fifth Point: COMMUNICATION

The next Point of Contact is located in the throat. Lower your chin toward your chest and press the back of your neck toward your partner, lifting your spine as you do. Relax your shoulders and press the backs of your shoulders into each other. Make a sound and feel the vibration of that sound flowing through both you and your partner. Imagine that the sound comes from a blue, glowing sphere in the throat and expands in waves in all directions, merging with the waves of your partner's blue sphere.

This is the Point of Contact related to communication. Take a moment to feel whatever is true for you at this time. Feel it without judgment or distortion, but with clear recognition of your truth. Imagine having that truth totally heard and understood by your partner. Open your consciousness to receiving your partner's truth without judgment or distortion, simply as a statement of what is so. Imagine that it's easy and effortless to share communication with your partner as you begin your practice. Allow the flow of communication to direct the flow of energy in a way that enhances your practice, by being willing to speak and listen to the truth.

Sixth Point: VISION

Next, bring your attention to the sixth Point of Contact, located between your eyes, two inches behind the front of the forehead. Keeping your eyes closed, bring your attention to the inner world of the third-eye center. At this point of contact we learn to see eye to eye with our partner and find our common vision.

Imagine a center of deep indigo blue glowing within your third eye. Imagine that this indigo glow is part of a divine light that illuminates the inside of your whole body. Imagine that a similar light dwells within your partner, filling his or her body. See this light expanding beyond the boundaries of your skins to merge into one light, radiating in all directions. See this light dissolving all illusions, bringing clarity and peace.

Even though your eyes are closed, open your psychic attention to really seeing your partner. See their beauty and radiance, their struggles and vulnerability. Imagine that you are two bodies of light intertwining and dancing together, each increasing the light of the other.

Seventh Point: UNION

Now bring your attention to the seventh Point of Contact, at the top of the head. This is the point that brings divine union between you and your partner, the ultimate goal of yoga. Feel the flow of energy rising up your spine from base to crown. Know that you can only feel this energy because there is a consciousness that is capable of that awareness. This consciousness pervades everything that is and you are part of that consciousness and it is part of you. Your divine gift is to share that awareness with your partner.

Imagine that the boundaries between you and your partner soften and completely dissolve, so that you become one being. Feel a larger awareness that is beyond the awareness within you or your partner yet encompasses you both. Allow yourself to surrender to that awareness, like a river surrendering to the sea.

Now imagine that each Point of Contact between you and your partner is glowing with aliveness and light, opening each center and expanding it into your partner. Your bodies are like two glowing rainbows, aligned and glowing with energy and awareness. Keep this awareness as you slowly begin to open your eyes and prepare for your practice.

part two

The SEVEN POINTS IN PRACTICE

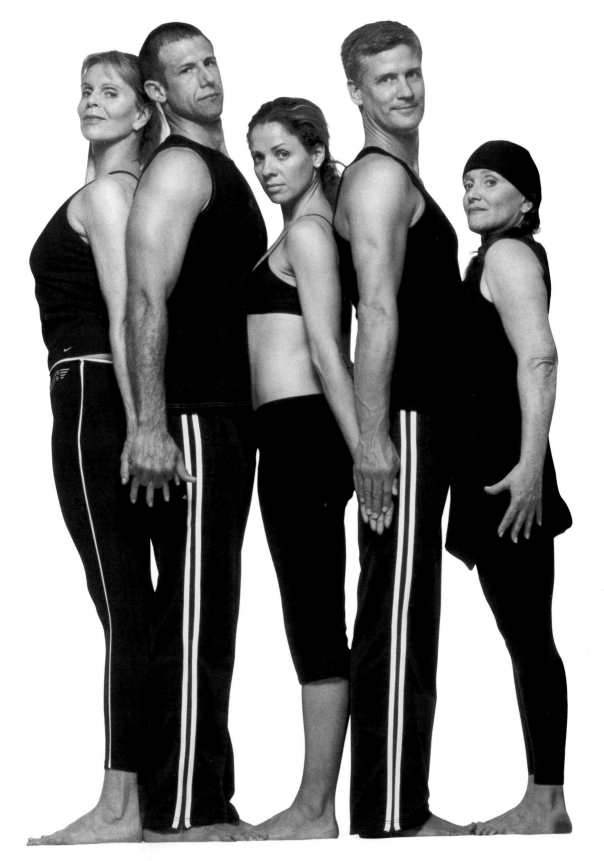

TRUST

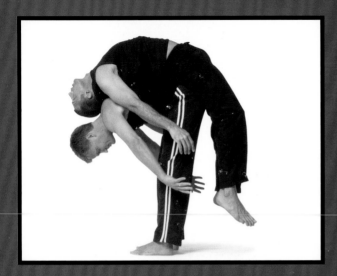

Qualities:

FOUNDATION
INTEGRITY
SECURITY

Gift:

SAFETY

Challenge:

FEAR

Relationship is a bridge built between two people. Across this bridge travel emotions and desires, dreams and aspirations, touches and treasures, as well as fears and insecurities— the countless little things that form the soul of any relationship. To take that vital risk to reach out to another person, you need a sense of trust. You want your love to be received, your words to be heard, your dreams to be embraced.

Bridges need a solid foundation. You need firm ground on which to build and the ability to reach beyond that ground to connect with another foundation on the other side. And you need roots into that ground. You need to know where you stand, even how to stand.

In Contact Yoga, as well as in relationship, the foundation is trust. This is our first Point of Contact, the place where everything begins. Without trust, nothing else can be sustained or even built. Again and again, every action will bring you back to this place. Without trust, you won't be able to "get off the ground" and move into deeper Contact. You won't be able to surrender to passion, make a commitment, open up to love, communicate clearly, see eye to eye, or find union. This first Point of Contact is utterly essential for all that is to come.

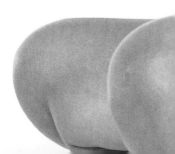

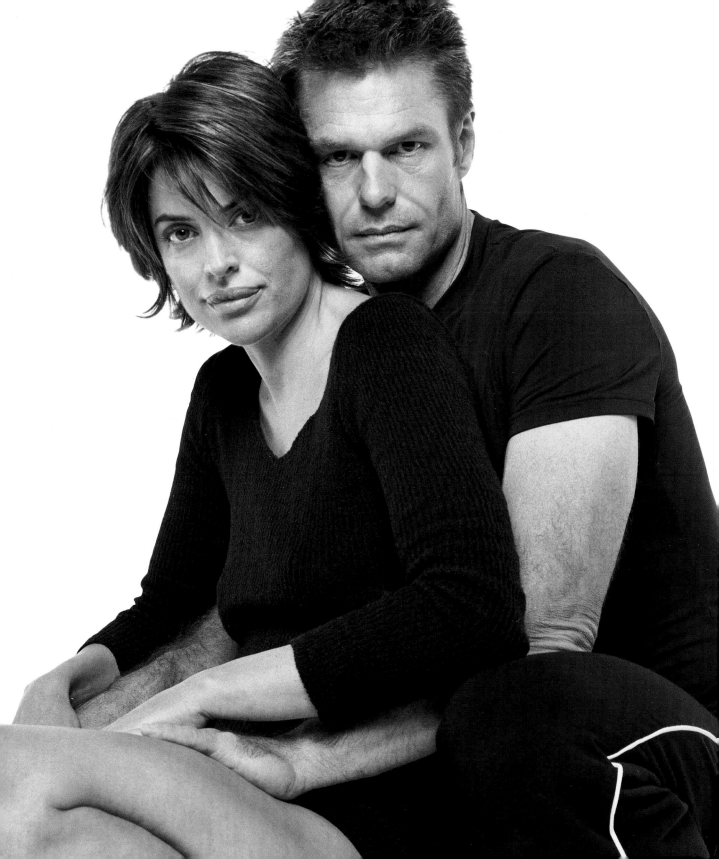

You need trust to feel a sense of security. A child feels this security through the mother's holding and touching. In Contact Yoga it occurs literally through making contact—not just with your hands, but also with your whole body, and not just your body, but with your emotions, intentions, desires, needs, offerings, and ideals. Only when these aspects are present and acknowledged can we deepen our trust and allow intimacy to blossom.

Trust cannot be granted; it must be earned. This takes time. Trust is built from consistency, solidity, and a continual willingness to be present and vulnerable, especially in the more difficult moments. It often arises out of little hurts that are then lovingly and compassionately mended, because by mending them, two people build a foundation together that will support their relationship. They form understandings, make agreements, learn about those vulnerable places in each other that need extra care and protection. Through stumbling across this bridge, you learn where you can trust your partner and where you can't.

Trust is about creating safety. In relationship, you can choose to be open and take risks when you know the odds are pretty good that it's safe to do so. In Contact, you can open deeply to a pose when you know you will be safely held. This takes practice and continual demonstration.

During this period of trust building, it's natural to test the ground of your partner—to see if it's really there, to find out if that ground can hold you in both your fears and your expansions. Make this testing into a game instead of a demand. Find a playful way of exploring together. Remove expectations, but communicate your needs.

It's easier to be playful if you have a sense of your own ground. Then you're not as dependent upon your partner to provide this ground for you, not as angry at your partner's imperfections. To have your own ground is to know where your center is, to know where you stand, to know what's important to you. In yoga, you find your center through strength and stability in your legs, which form the foundation of any pose. In Contact, that stability provides support for your partner as well.

Trust can also be betrayed. There are times when your partner fails to be there in the way you want them to be, when promises are broken and expectations are not met. Then trust gets eroded. Examine your expectations and see where you might be overextended. Then use the practices for this first Point of Contact to rebuild trust again in a playful, mutual way.

When trust is absent, it awakens fear, the challenge of this Point of Contact. Fear makes you shut down and hold back. Fear divides and separates. It draws the energy inward instead of outward. Fear makes the testing period into a serious issue rather than a playful episode. Fear creates a kind of desperation to have your partner behave a certain way *now*, and this spreads fear to your partner as well. That kind of pressure can make anyone withdraw. Wherever fear exists, we withdraw from contact, bodily and emotionally.

The antidote to fear is the constant building or rebuilding of trust. This happens through the body and in the first chakra. As you practice Contact Yoga, you will build trust by taking that daring risk to show your partner what you truly need and letting your body have the experience of being met, supported, and held. This requires communication, vision, commitment, and many of the other Points of Contact that we will be exploring.

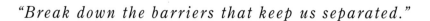

"Break down the barriers that keep us separated."

—*Tomas & Joan Hartfield, PhDs*

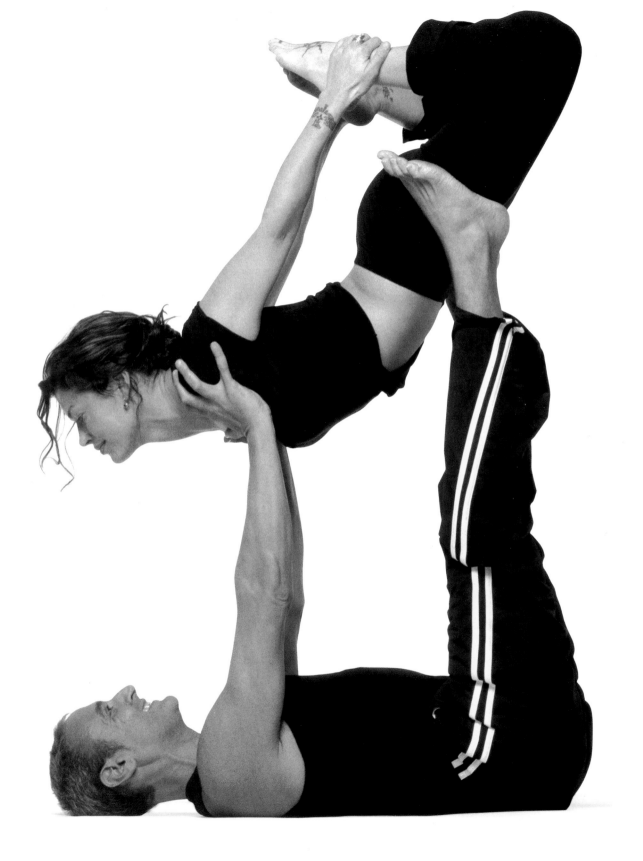

FLYING TRUST

GREG & STEPHEN

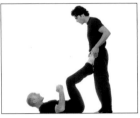

STEP 1 Greg places Stephen's feet along his outer hip/thigh crease.

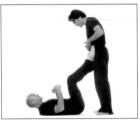

STEP 2 Greg and Stephen communicate to confirm that this is the right spot.

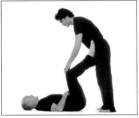

STEP 3 Maintaining eye contact, Greg leans forward.

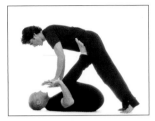

STEP 4 Stephen bends his knees to take Greg's weight over his center. He holds Greg's hands to help Greg balance.

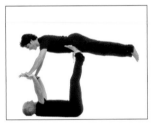

STEP 5 Palm to palm, Stephen moves his feet parallel as Greg extends his legs behind him.

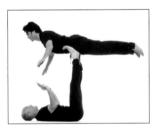

STEP 6 Stephen releases Greg's hands and uses his feet to help Greg balance.

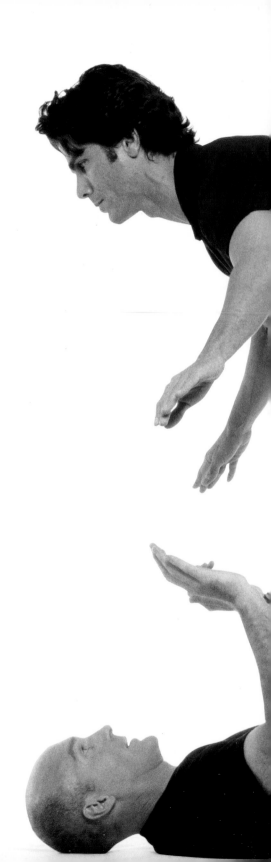

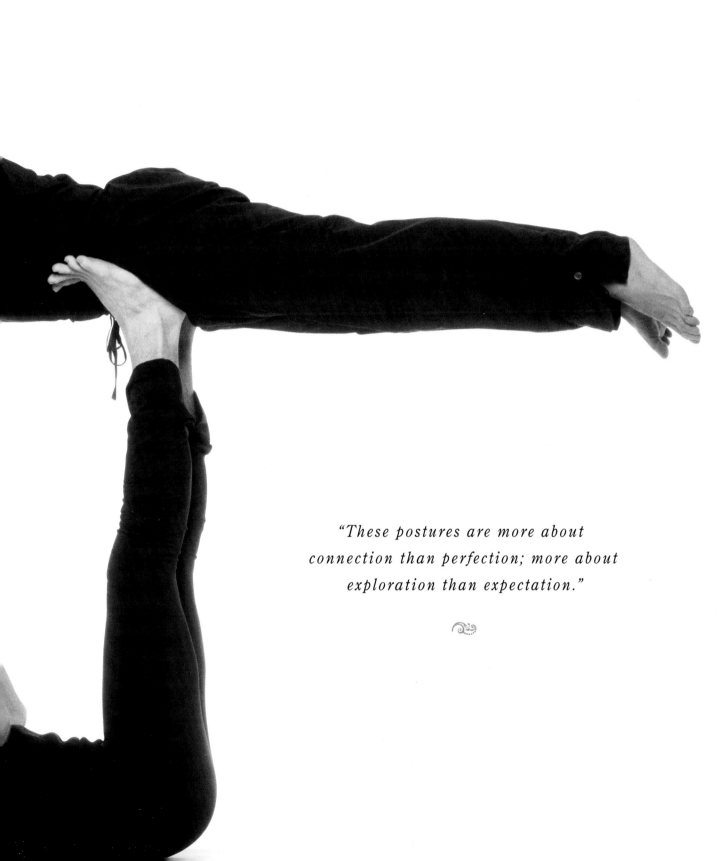

"These postures are more about connection than perfection; more about exploration than expectation."

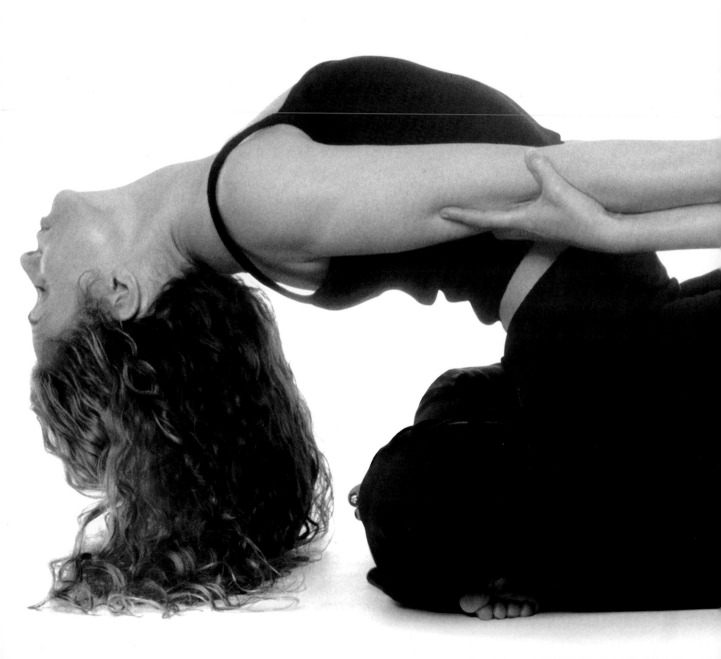

"It is important to note that Contact Yoga was born out of my inner intention and not my outward yoga practice."

—*Tara Guber*

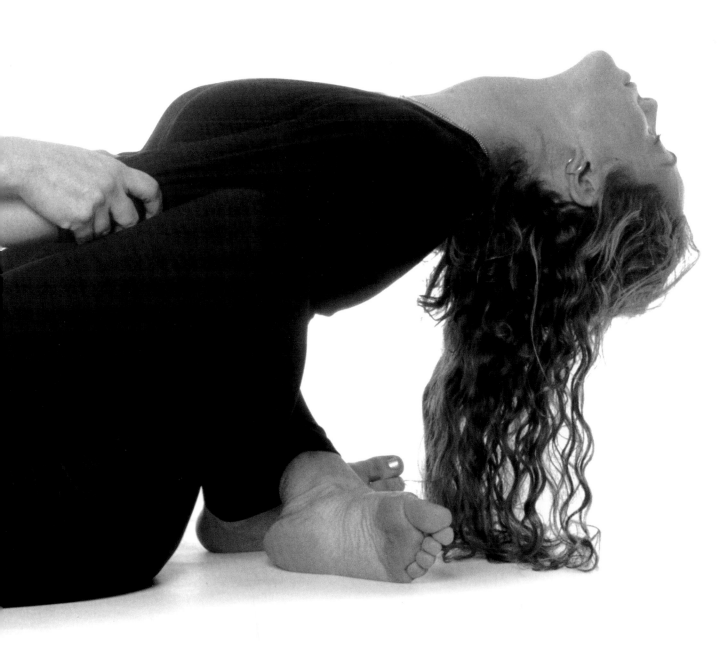

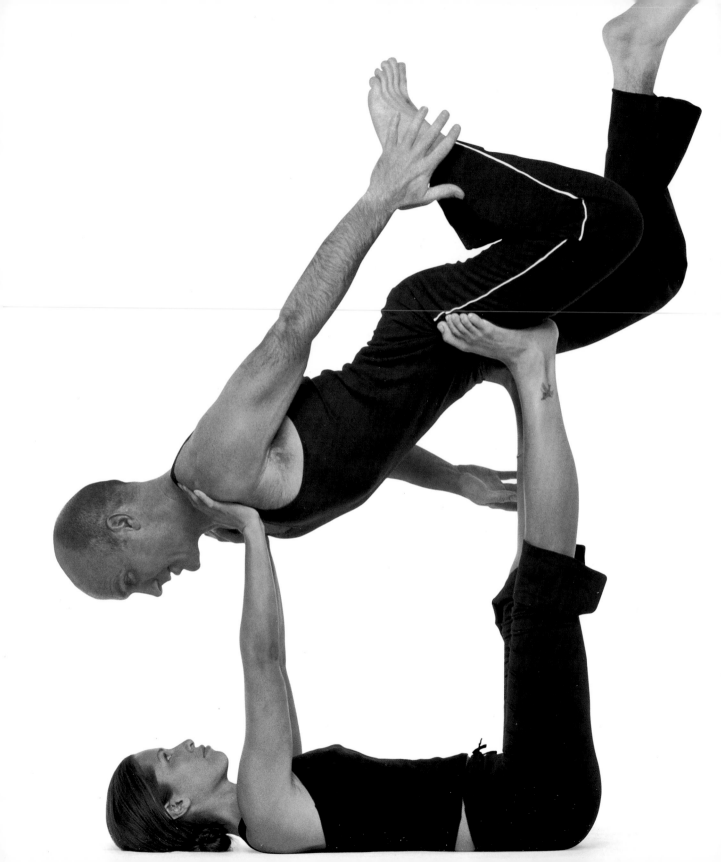

FLYING
STEPHEN & ELIZABETH

STEP 1 Elizabeth places Stephen's feet along her hip/thigh crease. Maintaining eye contact, Elizabeth leans forward.

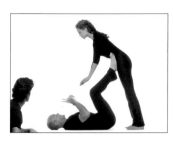

STEP 2 Stephen bends his knees to take Elizabeth's weight over his center. He holds Elizabeth's hands to help her balance.

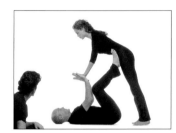

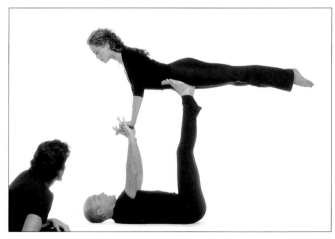

STEP 3 Palm to palm, Stephen presses his legs straight, and Elizabeth lifts off, extending her legs behind her. Trusting Stephen's support, Elizabeth flies!

"Silence speaks louder than words."

—*Baba Hari Dass*

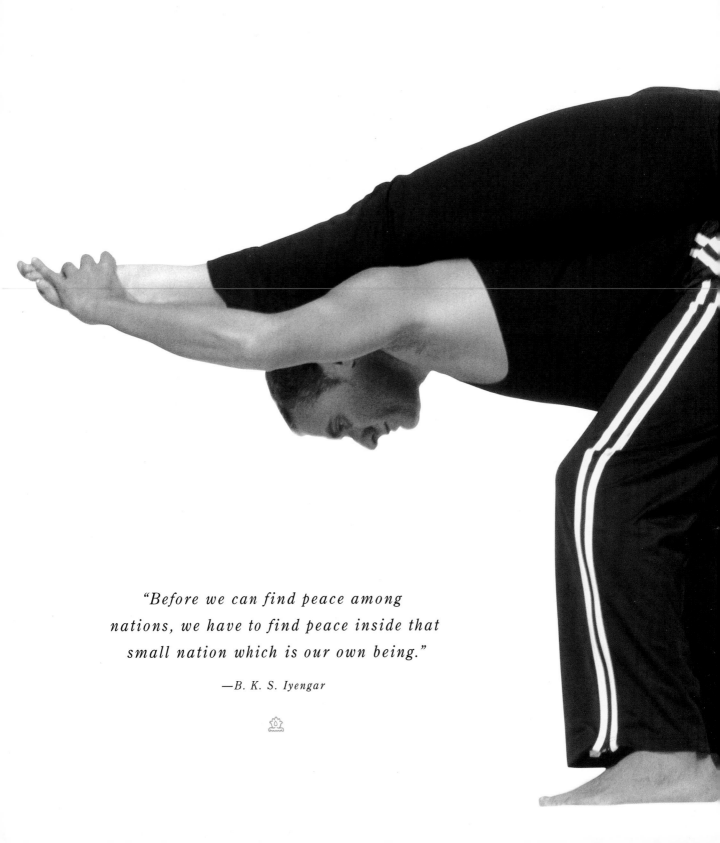

"Before we can find peace among
nations, we have to find peace inside that
small nation which is our own being."

—B. K. S. Iyengar

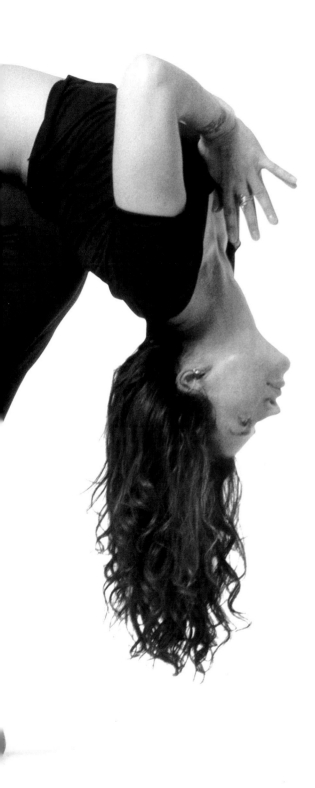

SPINAL ALIGNMENT
VINNIE & CARRÉ

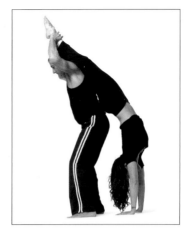

STEP 1 Carré does a handstand behind Vinnie's back. Vinnie catches her ankles and places his shoulders at the back of her knees.

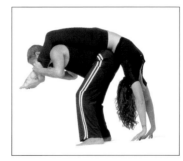

STEP 2 Vinnie hooks Carré's knees over his shoulders as he bends forward. Carré is lifted off her hands into a hanging backbend.

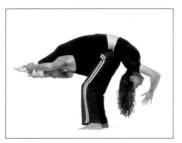

STEP 3 Vinnie lengthens his spine and arms as he pulls Carré's legs straight. Carré brings her hands into prayer.

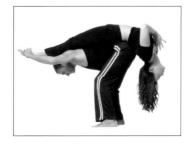

STEP 4 Vinnie arches his back, deepening the stretch. Carré brings her hands to her heart, in gratitude for this beautiful experience of opening through Contact.

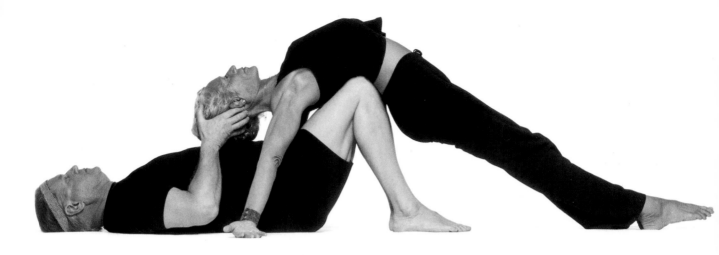

GUIDELINES FOR
TRUST IN PRACTICE

The first Point of Contact is based on the first chakra and its associated element, earth, the place where all foundations are built. This fundamental level relates to the body itself, the physicality of our flesh, its structure, its needs, indeed its very existence. All relationship involves bodies moving together in some way, sharing space, surviving together. The more contact those bodies have, and the more conscious we become about that contact, the deeper the relationship grows.

There is a powerful bonding in trying, failing, and trying again together until you succeed. As you work together over time, you learn about support—both giving and receiving—so you both can open enough to build this bridge of connection. How do you communicate trust to your partner, so they will be confident that you will really be there for them, while being there for yourself at the same time?

"As soon as you trust yourself, you will know how to live."

—*Johann Wolfgang von Goethe*

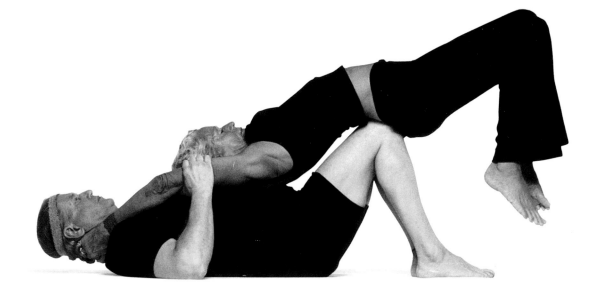

1. **FIND TRUST WITHIN YOURSELF.** Stay in your own ground at all times, keeping contact with your body and its sensations. Breathe in and listen to your inner voice. Only you truly know your limits, and you are the one responsible for protecting them.

2. **ESTABLISH SAFETY.** Honor your partner's body and its limitations and make sure your partner honors yours. Don't push yourself and don't let your partner push you. If your partner is new to yoga, or has a bad back or a weak knee, make sure you acknowledge these limitations, as well as express your own. Don't force your ideas of how a pose should go on your partner. Instead, be open to every part of the pose, every part of the experience. Find a way to make the pose work for you, at whatever angle you might be in, and feel how that can make it work for your partner as well. Trust your own process.

3. **GO SLOW.** Until you have practiced with someone for a while, you need to feel your way into a pose. When you move too fast, you miss many delicious moments of Contact. Alignment is more precise when you take your time. Allow for the hesitancy of newness. Remember, the goal at this first level is to make contact—nothing more, but also nothing less. Feel your way, gently, slowly, letting the body lead the mind.

4. **WORK YOUR LEGS.** Place your feet consciously, rooting down through your legs, making solid contact with the earth. Draw that solidity up into the body, holding your shape firmly, with determination. Because you are at times supporting another, this practice of rooting down is essential, and provides the strength you will need. If you are to win your partner's trust so they can truly surrender, you must learn to communicate that solid support through your flesh.

5. **USE YOUR WHOLE BODY.** Allow as much contact as possible, touching with hands, feet, backs, necks, bellies. Touch communicates that you are there with your partner. How much contact can you make with your bodies? How many square inches of skin can you put in contact with each other? How does that contact feel, and where does it take you?

6. **USE THE POSES** as a means of creating relatedness, not performance. If you slip out of yourself, you won't be able to be there for your partner. If you slip out of relatedness, you are missing the point. Reground yourself and start again; see where you slipped away.

7. **WHEN WORKING IN AREAS OF TRUST,** always try to move the energy downward. Become like two trees that are growing together, roots entwined, and reaching deep into the earth. Surrender to the feeling and mutual experience of trust in yourself and in others. If you doubt or are afraid, your partner probably shares that same feeling. Practice softening your body and mind, releasing resistance, and letting tension trapped in your body fall away.

PASSION

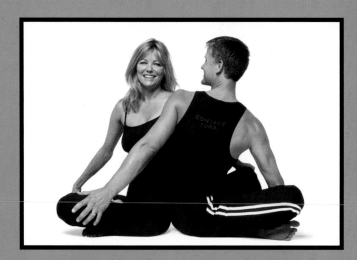

Qualities:

SENSUALITY
PLEASURE
DESIRE

Gift:

JOY

Challenge:

SURRENDER

The second Point of Contact connects us with the essence of life itself: the power of passion. With all the force of a rushing river, passion carries us beyond our habitual limitations. Here we flow with the primordial energy of life, the very energy that drives us to create life. When you approach Contact with passion, enthusiasm, and excitement, you open yourself to this powerful, regenerative energy.

Passion, as the focus of our second Point of Contact, relates to the second chakra, located in the sacral area. The energy of this chakra can be repressed by fear, anxiety, rejection, abuse, or any important experience you may have had as a child or adult. But when allowed to flow freely, passion opens that river of excitement that leads to joy. Passion is courted by pleasure and rooted in sensuality, flowing through the watery realms of emotion with all its needs and desires. Once trust is established, passion invites you to go to the next step.

To face your partner with openness and vulnerability may seem overwhelming at times. If it were not for passion, we probably wouldn't do it at all. Passion makes us want to be there, in body, mind, and spirit. Passion drives us to show up.

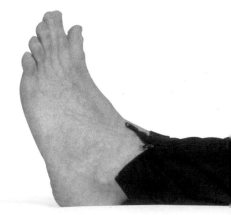

*"Through the eyes of truth,
integrity, and passion,
relating becomes sublime."*

—*Margot Anand*

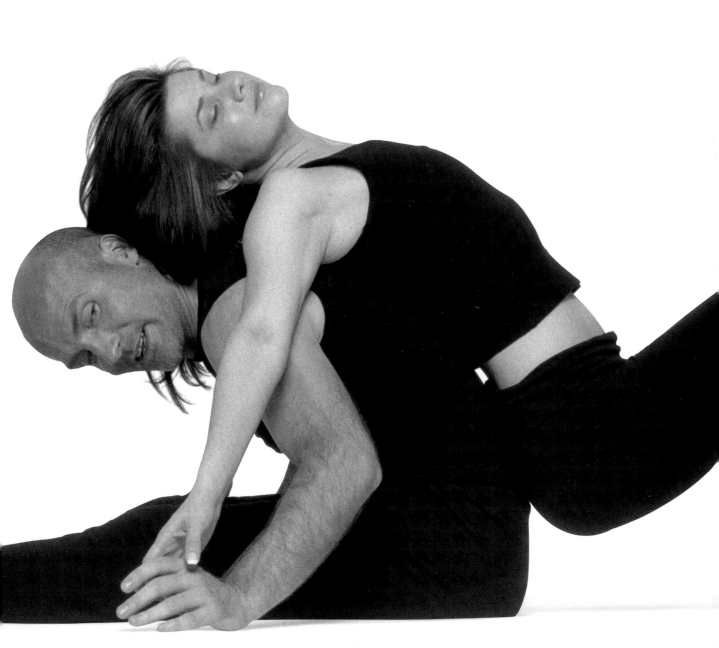

But whether you practice Contact with a long-term partner or a fellow student you just met, opening to passion is essential. It will bring you deeper into the rivers of your vital energy and enhance the degree to which you are present for yourself, your partner, and your experience together.

Passion is a prime motivator, whether it's about a project, an idea, or a partner. In keeping with the second Point's element of water, pleasure and passion make life juicy. Without them, life becomes too intellectual, dull, and dry. Through pleasure, the rivers of feeling within each partner flow deeply and become one, creating an ocean of heightened awareness.

One of the greatest challenges in a long-term relationship is to keep that Passion alive throughout the ups and downs of the daily grind. Few relationships survive—or even begin—without passion. How else would we overcome the fear of intimacy and all its risks? The key is bringing more passion into your life and practice.

Maybe you're not sure how to do that. Maybe you think it requires something beyond your capabilities, or fear that you might be rejected, or that it's going to take more work than you are prepared to invest. If so, you won't get very far, because none of these concepts make it very inviting.

But when you approach Contact with an attitude of playful vitality and excitement and allow the currents of passion to carry you, it becomes sheer delight, a stimulating adventure that's easy and fun. Let go of goals and expectations, and enter into the delicious moment of now. Let go of the chatter in your head and drop down into your sensate experience. At this Point of Contact, your body's sensations will be your ultimate guide.

Surrender is the gateway to passion, yet it is also the challenge. To do so, we must be willing to surrender the safety of the known to enter the unknown. If we choose to resist—out of fear or the desire to control—we diminish the mystery that is calling us forth.

The challenge of surrender is to maintain our center in those first waves of excitement and not drown in the white water of passion. When the roots of trust are strong, we may safely surrender to passion without losing our ground, allowing the momentum of the energy flow to build.

Pleasure makes things feel good and invites us to repeat the experience. Pleasure also invites love, requires communication, inspires vision, and smoothes the way for union and bliss. Pleasure, when poured like the waters of the second Point onto the roots of trust, helps the relationship grow toward Commitment, the next Point of Contact.

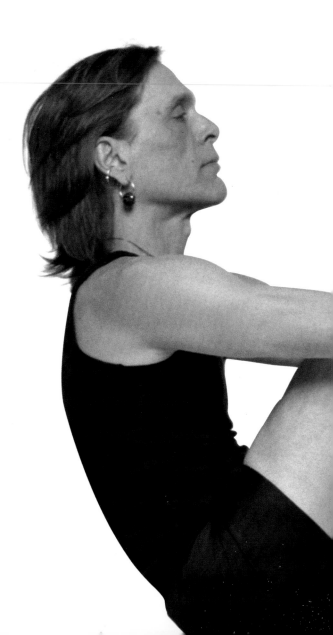

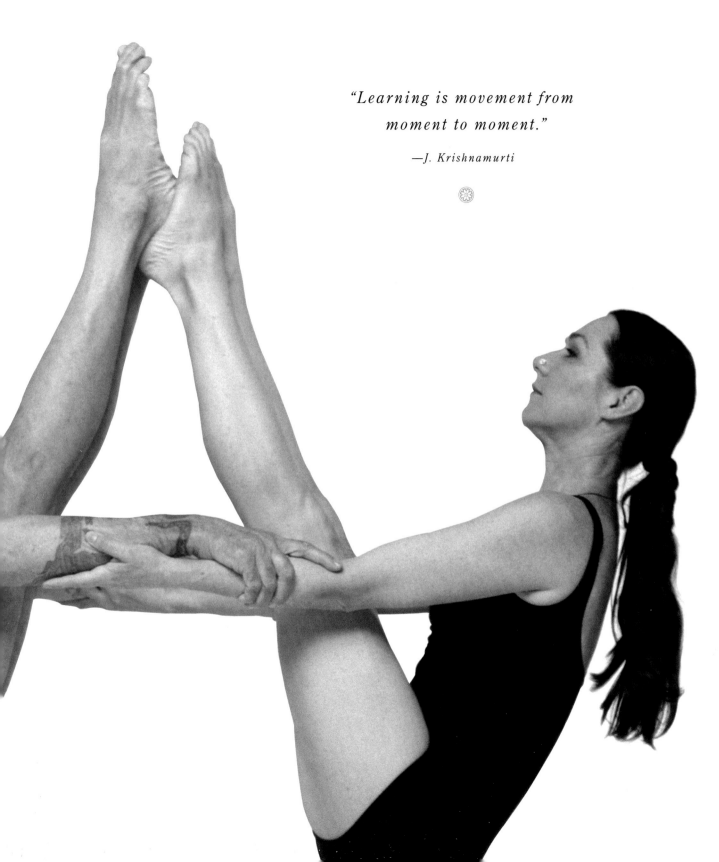

"*Learning is movement from moment to moment.*"

—*J. Krishnamurti*

The MEETING of
SHIVA & SHAKTI

In the Hindu system of deities, Shiva and Shakti intertwine in a constant state of divine passion, representing the eternal regenerating forces of the universe. They also represent the universal polarities within us all: Shiva, the limitless force of pure consciousness; and Shakti, the primordial energy of creation. When Shiva and Shakti unite, Shiva gives form to Shakti's raw potential. Their union creates all levels of manifestation and realization of the eternal state of being in the heart.

Shiva and Shakti first meet in Anahata, the place of the heart. Shiva, residing in the crown, is content and dreaming in his own dominion, being both part regent of all he surveys.

Shakti calls to Shiva, saying, "Awake, my lord, and descend into life with me. Trust me, my lord, I am only here for our union and for your highest dreams; please believe that your dreams are also mine.

"Within me lies your own fulfillment as well as the resolution of your fears of departing from the luxury and comfort of your own heaven. Through me lies the path of your own transformation.

"If you do not believe me, you will remain, dreaming forever, in the realm of heaven. If you choose not to manifest in creation, do not answer my call. If you are not going to become all that you are destined to be, choose to stay asleep."

And hearing her, Shiva chooses to answer her call.

Chakra by chakra, she pulls him down from his head and his heart, down from his intellect and idealism. She is joined by her dark sister, the raging and sexual Kali, who arouses Shiva from his slumber and brings him into the fiery core of his resistance and fear.

Through the fire and passion of Kali and with the loving and wise guidance of Shakti, Shiva finds his home in Shakti and through her is fully realized and fulfilled. It is from their union that all of creation forever flows.

When allowed to flow safely, passion brings the gift of joy. Nectar from the gods, the sharing of joy is a potent sacrament, a nourishing drink that sweeps energy into the upper chakras, opening the heart and leading to union and grace.

"Contact Yoga is an external expression of an internal union based on sacred relationship."

—Ken "Tesh" Scott

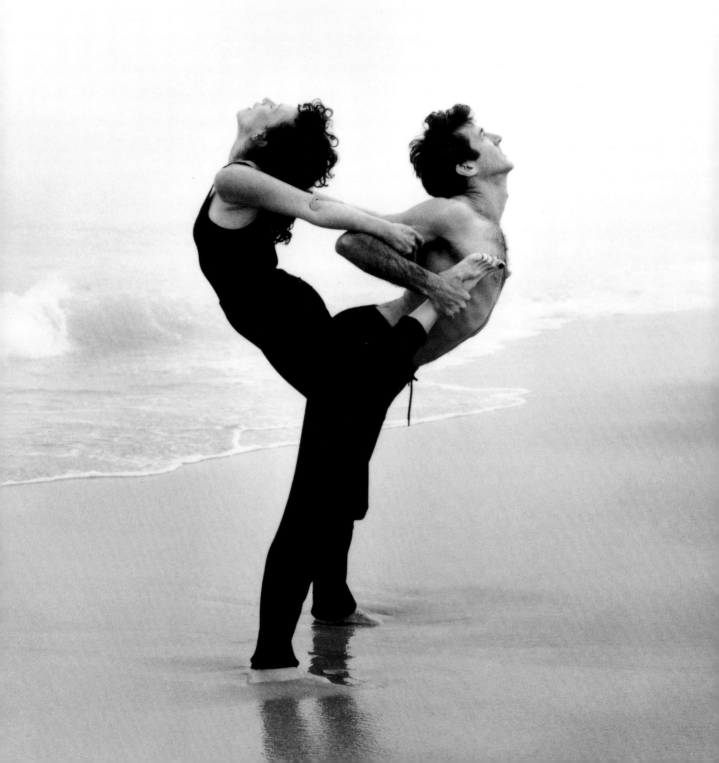

GUIDELINES FOR
PASSION IN PRACTICE

It's important to state here that the experience of passion by two partners in Contact is not by definition sexual. As in all yoga, Contact evokes, expresses, and exchanges energy. This vital energy excites, inspires, delights, and restores not only your practice but also all aspects of your life and relationships. It is the responsibility of each partner to recognize and channel this energy, to be responsible and appropriate at all times in its expression with your Contact partner or within your relationship.

The best way to remain faithful to your practice is to make it rewarding and fulfilling. When you encounter pleasure and delight in an experience, it doesn't take a lot of convincing to do it again. Pleasure is an invitation to do something again and again.

If Contact Yoga is a dynamic dance between two people, then touch is the music that orchestrates that dance. It awakens your kinesthetic sense, the oldest part of your brain. If you're going to move, touch is a way to get you going. It orients you to your body, and sensation orients your body to the world. Even if you don't know your partner well, touch is a way of saying hello—to yourself as you receive and to another as you reach out to connect.

Many people are touchy about touch. Our culture teaches us to distrust touch as something that may signal unwanted sexual contact. Consequently, we learn to hold back our own impulses to touch and hold back from contact as well. If you are practicing with a partner you don't know very well, take a few moments to explore any issues you have about touch. Express what makes you uncomfortable in giving or receiving touch and share any fears you may have. Also, express the kind of touch you especially like or want. This helps deepen the trust and allows the opening of passion to happen safely.

Touch has its own conversation. You reach out to caress, and your partner responds. The conversation flows back and forth like lines of poetry, dancing in sensual communion. To feel another's touch upon your skin is the most primal language there is. It is the first language of a child, the only way infants can know they are safe and loved.

Have you ever felt the kind of touch that speaks to your very soul? Can you feel the warmth that surrounds you in the arms of someone you love? What does it call forth from you, and how do you respond? If you're like most people, it helps you let down your barriers, dissolve your boundaries, and settle deep into the body. It signals (whether it's true or not) that everything's going to be okay.

That's because touch produces endorphins, the natural opiates of the body that are an antidote to pain and produce euphoria. But that's not all. When your skin is stroked, it produces an important peptide called oxytocin, the chemical that makes you want to form relationships, to bond, and to make contact. After a while, just thinking of your lover can make your oxytocin level spike. This creates the longing to be together in that altered state of consciousness that makes you feel you can't live without him or her, and that horrible feeling of withdrawal when you're apart. But while oxytocin makes you want to bond, it also hazes the mind into forgetfulness, which is why a mother forgets the pain of childbirth. It's why touch is so important for softening anger after a fight, and may explain why some people bond with inappropriate partners, forgetting their drawbacks. Touch is so essential for a relationship to thrive that without it couples become alienated. Touch is the great healer that reaches across distance and brings intimacy.

*"We can create an alliance that
allows us to actually use our mind
rather then be used by it."*

—*Sakyong Mipham Rinpoche*

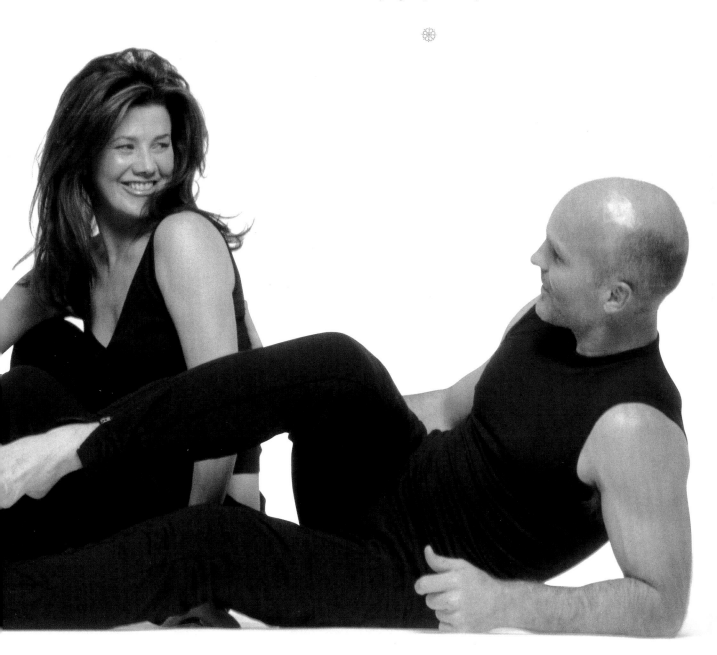

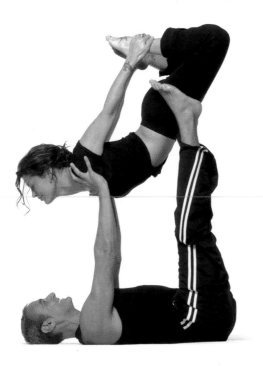

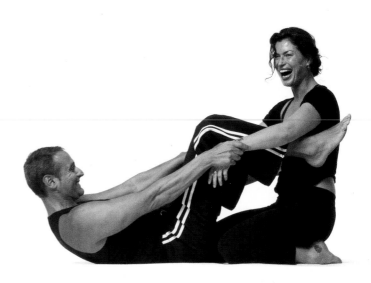

1. **ESTABLISH YOUR CONTACT THROUGH TOUCH.** Before trying any of the poses, take turns learning to receive touch. Close your eyes and let your partner tune into your emotional body through his or her hands. Make contact with the one that lives inside as you feel from deep within your soul. If you are the one receiving, give your partner feedback, with both abstract sound and with words: "Ooh, that feels good," "A little softer here, and a little more over there." Be playful with each other. Make it into a game that has no goal other than the pleasure of connection in the moment.

2. **EMBRACE YOUR EMOTIONAL BODY** and bring it forth to your partner. As you touch with hands, eyes, spines, bellies, or feet, drop down into your flesh and into your feelings. You

might show your feelings with words, sound, movement, a look, or a caress: allow your emotions to fill the sensate cells of the body as you work and play together. Like an invisible guide, emotional rapport will develop and help to deepen the experience of each move you make together. Let your emotional streams flow together.

3. **HAVE A TOUCH CONVERSATION WITH YOUR PARTNER.** Just as we use words to express our internal feelings to each other, listen to your partner's response and then speak again. See how eloquently you can converse with your touch. Let your hand say something to your partner, without words. Let your partner respond with a touch. Let the conversation flow back and forth, feeling your way for several minutes.

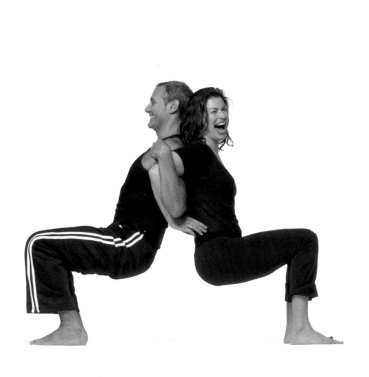

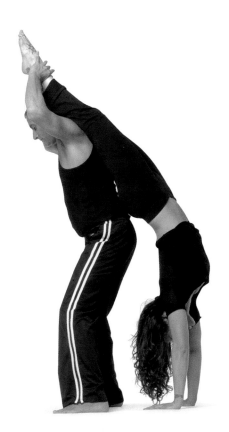

4. **APPLY THIS SAME CONCEPT TO YOUR WHOLE BODY.** Once your touch conversation begins to be reciprocal, then you have the basic language with which to speak with your body. Be playful, expressive, and creative. Use your body as if it were a hand, reaching, receiving, caressing. Let your partner respond with his or her own movement, continuing the conversation until both your bodies feel engaged in the contact.

5. **CHANNEL THE EROTIC ENERGY BUILT THROUGH CONTACT.** These poses can be very sensuous, and the erotic energy can be very intoxicating. Take this energy and focus it, enliven it, and honor it. Use this passion as a kind of fuel that is not specifically sexual: for some, it can be even more intimate than sexual contact. If you don't want to be sexual, if you're with a partner you don't know well, for example, then allow this energy to travel through your own body as an increased form of aliveness.

6. **LAUGH, PLAY, AND HAVE FUN TOGETHER.** Bring pleasure into your practice, and follow your passions together. This is spirituality at its best: joyful, delightful, and powerful.

> *"We are like islands in the sea, separated on the surface but connected in the deep."*
>
> —*William James*

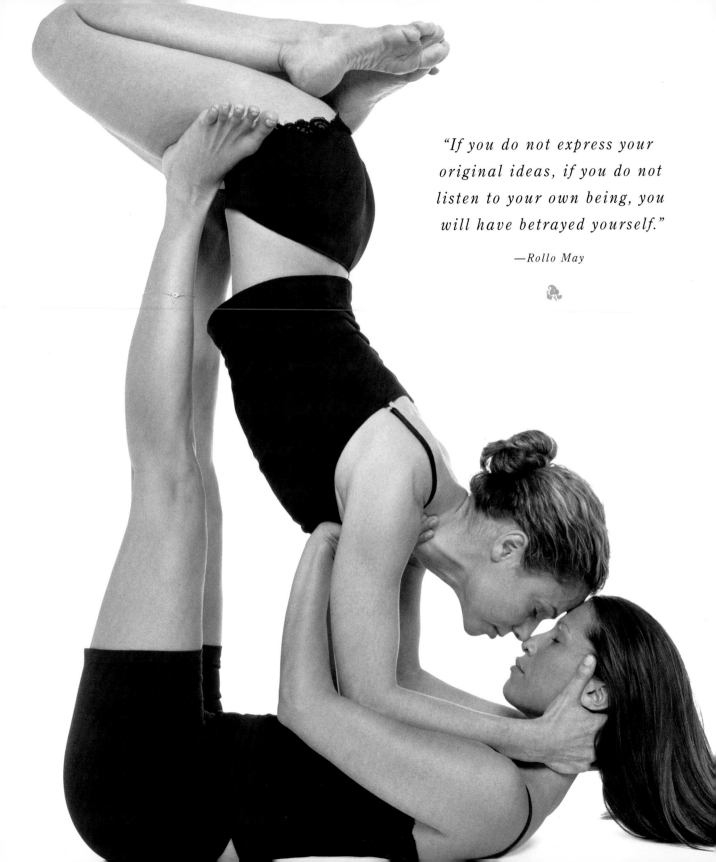

"If you do not express your original ideas, if you do not listen to your own being, you will have betrayed yourself."

—Rollo May

HANGING

SEANE & RAINBEAU

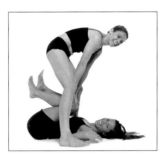

STEP 1 Seane and Rainbeau playfully prepare—Seane on top and Rainbeau below.

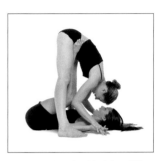

STEP 2 They slow their breathing, center themselves, and make contact. Rainbeau places her feet in Seane's groin. Seane releases into a forward bend and they interlace fingers.

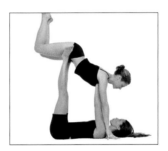

STEP 3 Rainbeau straightens her legs, lifting Seane into flying. She places her hands on Seane's shoulders for upper-body support. Seane presses her fingertips into the floor to lengthen her back and open her heart.

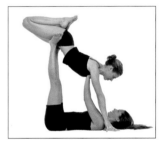

STEP 4 Seane bends at the knees, bringing her feet to her buttocks.

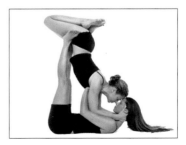

STEP 5 Seane clasps her hands behind Rainbeau's neck. They touch their foreheads together, coming into union.

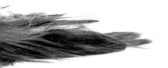

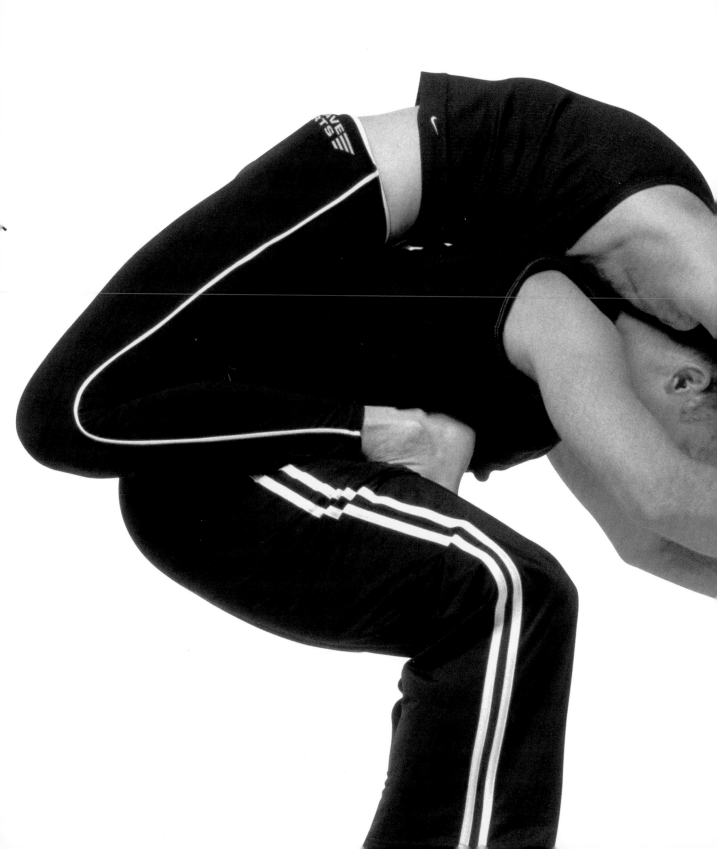

BACK PACK
PATRICIA & JULES

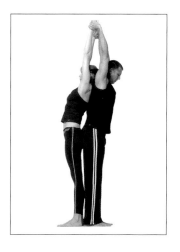

STEP 1 Patricia and Jules stand back-to-back. Jules places his feet shoulder width apart. They reach for contact all along their spines, synchronizing their breath.

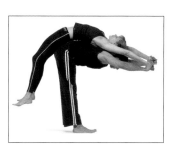

STEP 2 Once they have established trust through the communication of their breath, Jules slowly bends forward and gently lifts Patricia into a backbend, allowing their sacra to connect.

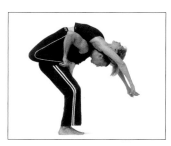

STEP 3 Patricia surrenders into the backbend as Jules places her feet over his thighs.

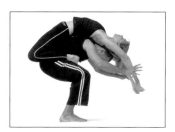

STEP 4 Jules holds Patricia's wrists. As he arches his back, he gently pulls her arms to stretch her spine as he begins to squat down.

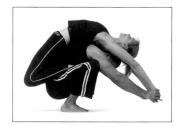

STEP 5 Jules goes into full squat as Patricia breathes, and surrenders into a deep backbend.

EXTENDED BACKBEND

BAHNI & STEPHEN

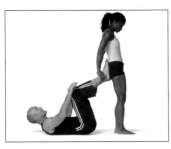

STEP 1 Bahni arranges Stephen's feet on her sacrum and buttocks so they feel comfortable. They breathe and feel their connection through touch, establishing trust through communication before continuing.

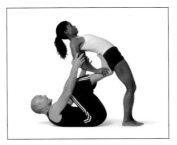

STEP 2 When ready, Bahni holds Stephen's ankles and leans back over his feet. Stephen supports her, holding her upper arms and guiding her backward.

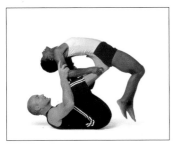

STEP 3 When Bahni is in full backbend, Stephen checks in to make sure his feet are in the right place and she feels safe.

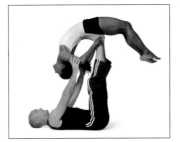

STEP 4 Stephen presses his legs straight to lift Bahni into a backward flying position, holding her upper arms firmly.

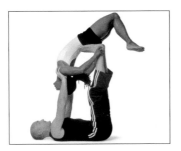

STEP 5 Stephen's hands move to Bahni's shoulders. Bahni communicates with Stephen physically and/or verbally about the angle of his feet so that they continue to support her deepening backbend. Bahni places her hands on Stephen's chest, as Stephen supports Bahni with his hands and feet to help her flip her legs over and bring her feet to the floor.

"Nothing great in the world has been accomplished without passion."

—*Georg Wilhelm Friedrich Hegel*

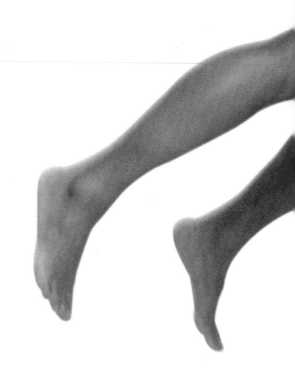

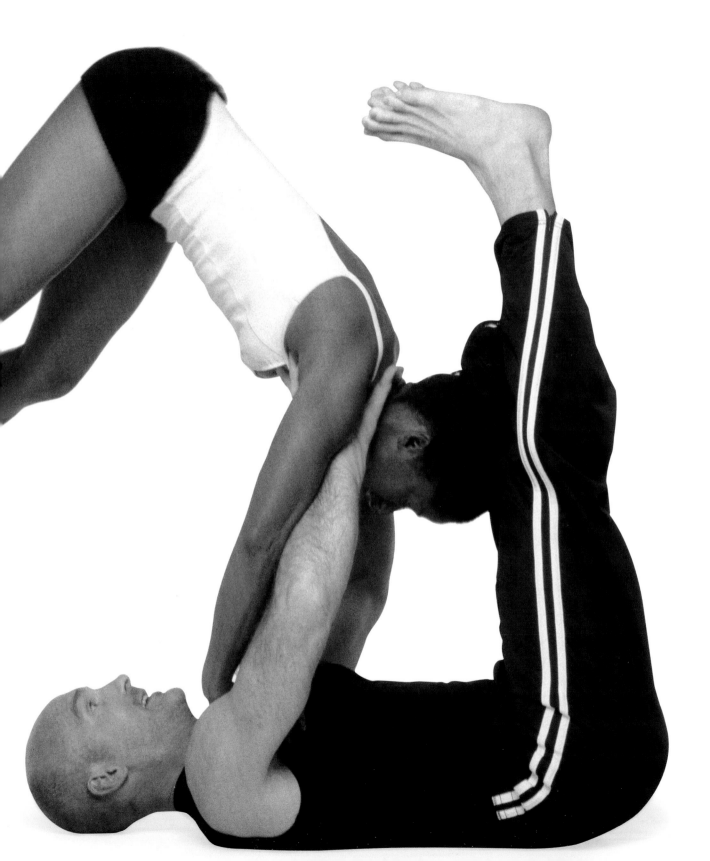

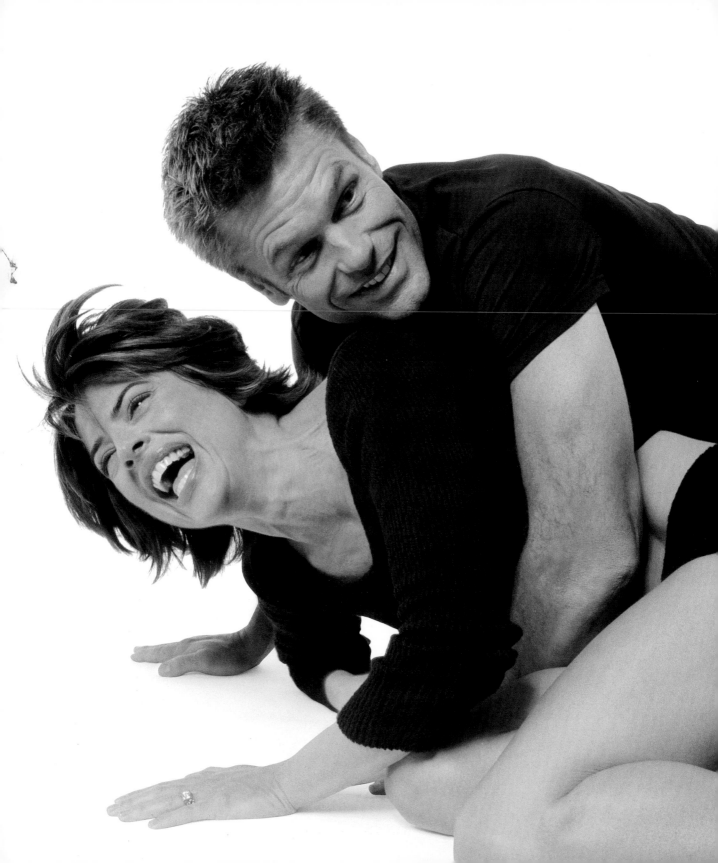

*"The most wasted of all days
is one without laughter."*

—*e. e. cummings*

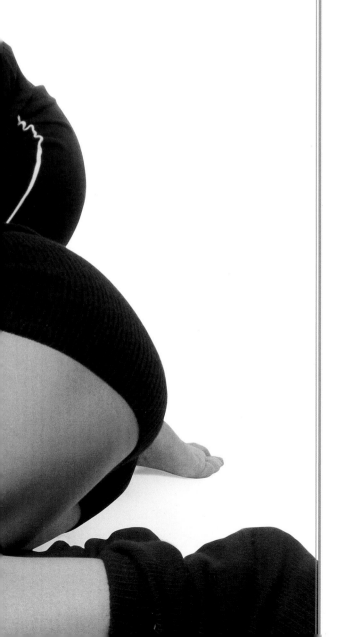

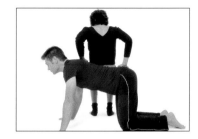

STEP 1 Harry gets on hands and knees in table position. Lisa squats at Harry's side, arching gently over his back. (She does not sit on his back!)

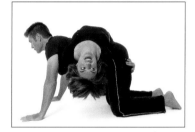

STEP 2 Lisa lies backward over Harry. She reaches her arms under his torso to hook around his thigh and shoulder. Harry arches and flexes his back like a cat.

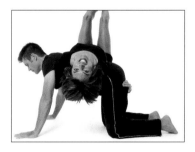

STEP 3 Bracing herself with her arms around Harry, Lisa lifts both legs.

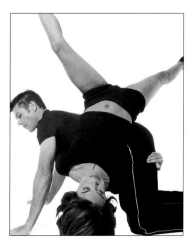

STEP 4 Harry holds steady as Lisa shifts to stretch her legs wide.

COMMITMENT

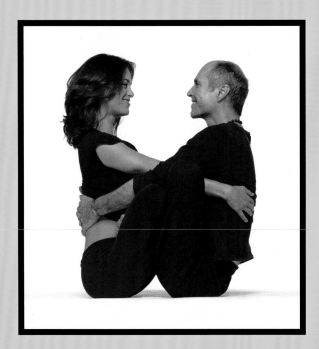

Qualities:

WILL

DISCIPLINE

RESPONSIBILITY

Gift:

FREEDOM

Challenge:

STRUGGLE

If you follow the river of passion, it eventually leads you into deeper water, yielding a new perspective and calling for new skills. It no longer carries you so easily, but requires your added effort to remain buoyant in a greater and deeper sea.

In any new venture, whether a relationship, a practice, or a business, your passion will eventually lead you to the testing moment of commitment. Passion brings you to the door; commitment determines whether you walk through it. But if you want to reach the next level, walk through you must.

Commitment is a conscious choice to achieve something deeper. It honors the sacred by creating a vessel of protection that supports growth. It channels creative energy into new pathways instead of allowing it to randomly disperse.

Commitment requires the intentional dedication of your energy—not just once, but over and over again. Here, the elemental fires of your third chakra forge two energies into one power. Instead of following the waters of the second Point of Contact wherever they might go, this third Point of Contact works on building the banks of the river, directing the energy toward a mutually chosen goal. This is no small thing, and it doesn't happen overnight.

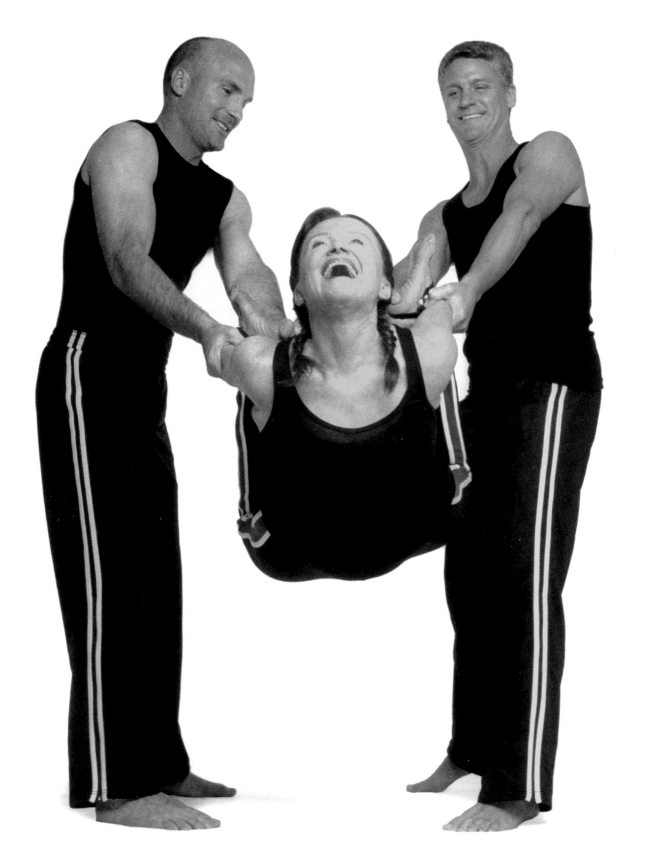

Commitment is one of the most challenging aspects of relationship. What happens when you make a commitment? Do you feel afraid that you will be too confined? Do you relax into complacency? Do you force your partner into commitment as a replacement for trust? What if your partner wants more commitment than you do, or wants it before you are ready? Do you commit from a place of obligation and duty?

Maybe you wonder if your partner is going to stick around. Maybe you're not sure whether you want to stick around. Maybe things are good with your partner, but you're not sure if they're good enough. Maybe they're so good you can't believe it will last and you push for commitment too soon. How do we get past this "make it or break it" fluctuation in the flow of a relationship? How do we sort through the issues of committing ourselves without the fear of losing ourselves?

In relationship, the concept of commitment comes with a lot of baggage. Some people crave it, while others run from it. Some think it brings security, while others see it as a trap, waiting to snare you in its teeth and swallow you whole.

But commitment need not be a blanket agreement to obligation. Instead, it can be a process of directing energy that creates freedom. You can choose what you want to commit to and choose it consciously. You can choose what you want to avoid and make that part of your commitment as well. You can set your intentions for your relationship and for your practice to be anything that is mutually desired. When commitment is given as a full-bellied act of will, it enlivens and intensifies the energy both within you and between you and your partner.

It's important to remain conscious of the intention behind commitment. Some people say they are committed to a relationship just because their physical body comes home every night, because they're not fantasizing about leaving, or because they do pretty well at keeping their agreements. This is an outer commitment, but it might not be a commitment of real presence, of energy, and of the transformational fires of the will. This deeper, energetic commitment forms a crucible for the creative and rejuvenating fires of the relationship to actually forge a path to freedom and bliss. You can commit to showing up for whatever contact you have—in the present moment or during practice—even if outer commitments are not formed.

If you and your partner have created enough trust and passion to enter more deeply into your relationship, sooner or later you'll encounter a clash of wills. You may want to do things one way; your partner may want another way. Here begins the challenge of this Point; the struggle that can bind the vital energy between you. In struggle there is friction; heat is created and the fires of the third Point are ignited. Heat can fuse two things into one if it is channeled appropriately. Struggle can make or break your relationship. When commitment is strong, struggle gives way to resolution, and the energy flows without distraction or obstruction. The gift of this resolution is freedom, which harvests the energy of the struggle and lets us move forward. We accept our commitment to the practice, to each other, or to a vision, and this containment allows the energy to build.

Transformation and mastery are the rewards of the third Point of Contact—essential elements in any yoga. This leads into even deeper contact and begins forging the vessel for the next Point of Contact, which is love.

"To be a warrior is to learn to be genuine in every moment of your life."

—*Chogyam Trungpa Rinpoche*

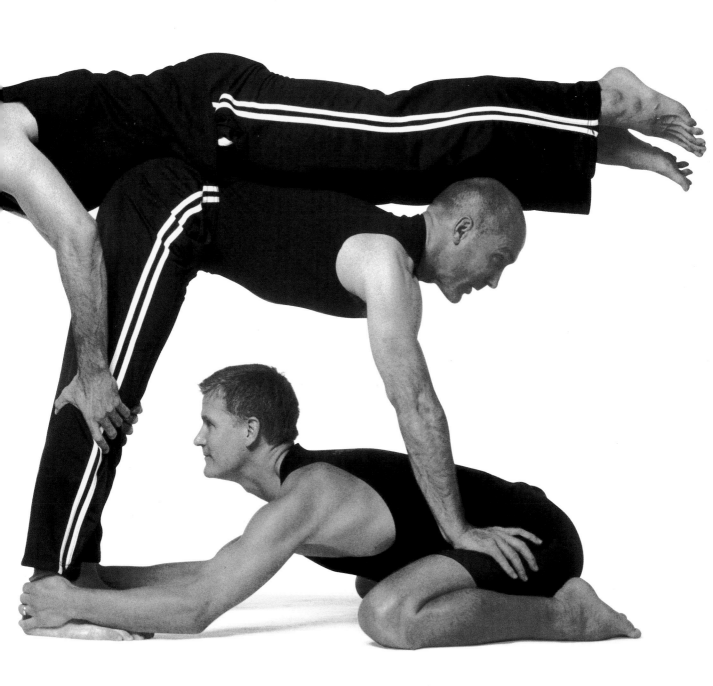

GUIDELINES FOR
COMMITMENT IN PRACTICE

It is miraculous that two distinct beings, each with their own will, manage to coordinate their power at all. It helps to have a form in which to channel and align energies. Repeated practice of Contact Yoga provides that form by creating context with our bodies so the inner fires have a place to flow.

The best things in life take time. The fruits of your practice are harvested only when cultivated by time and discipline, repeated focus and effort, dedication and honoring. To eventually find union–the true goal of yoga–your moves must be coordinated

with your partner's by repeated practice, so that you go beyond thought and enter fully into the flow of two beings becoming one.

When we invoke pleasure in the second Point of Contact, we court an element that invites us to "show up"–to be present. But not everything in a relationship is pleasurable. And in any spiritual practice, there are places along the way that are far less inviting than others, places where pleasure alone will not carry us through.

This is when we have to show up in our bodies by sheer force of will. We do this by filling our bodies with energy, asserting our strength in a pose, and holding solidity in our form. We do this by first finding that power in ourselves, by learning to hold our own shape in the face of adversity.

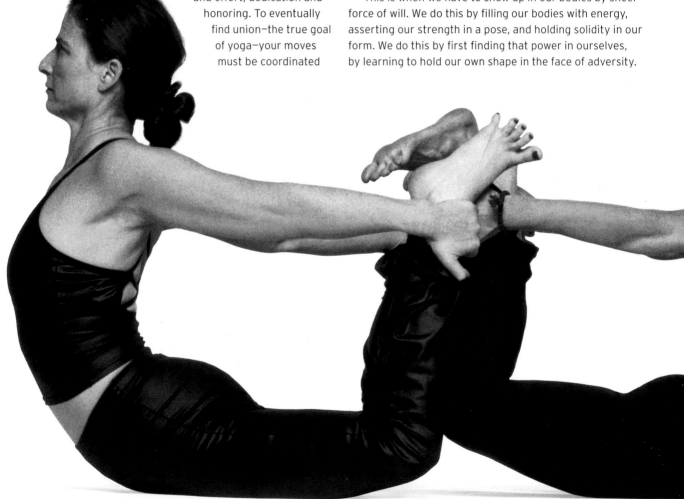

> *"One of life's greatest risks is never daring to risk."*
>
> —*Oprah Winfrey*

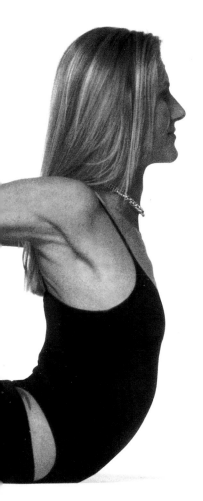

COMMITMENT
EXERCISE

T ake a simple standing pose of any variety, standing with your energy rooted through your legs, feet wide enough apart to keep your balance when challenged, bending the knees enough to give you some flexibility. Allow your partner to lean his or her weight against you without shifting your form. Don't be rigidly defended; allow yourself to meet your partner, but keep your own stance firm and strong. See what it feels like to both you and your partner when you remain steadfast and unflinching. Switch roles and experience the reverse side of this dynamic. Then share your experiences with each other.

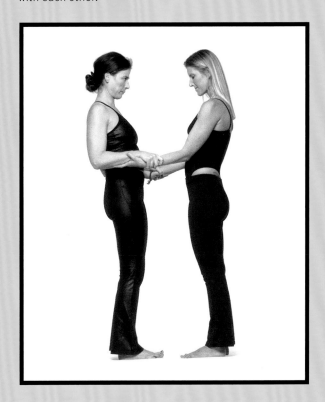

1. **MAKE A COMMITMENT TO YOUR PRACTICE.** Whether it's every morning, Tuesday afternoons, or once a month, empower yourself by making and keeping a commitment to practice together. This will be a time for your relationship to grow and for you to be together, as well as a time for you to work your body.

2. **PUT YOUR BODY ON THE LINE.** Learn what it means to show up. Commit with your movements, your intention, your strength, and your support. Commit to moving as fully as possible into each pose. Commit to repeating moves you have practiced and commit to at least one thing that is new each time: a different way of doing a pose or a different attitude toward your partner.

3. **REFINE YOUR COMMITMENTS.** Decide what you want to commit to and make it clear what you want to avoid. If you commit to an amount of time for your practice, stick to it, but don't commit for longer periods than you can handle. Be realistic. In your relationship, differentiate between the commitments you feel ready to make and the ones that are too confining.

4. **MAKE COMMITMENT AN ACT OF HONORING.** Honor first your needs, your fears, and your goals, and then honor your partner's needs, fears, and goals. Honor the person who stands before you and commit to being fully present with them during your practice.

5. **STATE YOUR COMMITMENTS.** Pick simple things: I commit to showing up. I commit to being strong enough for you. I commit to having fun. I commit to exploration. I commit to pleasing you. I commit to being there for myself.

6. **FEEL YOUR COMMITMENT AS AN ENERGIZING FIRE.** Enjoy it, surrender to it, and embody it. Allow it to strengthen you, to give you confidence. Allow it to increase trust and passion, and form a glowing container for love.

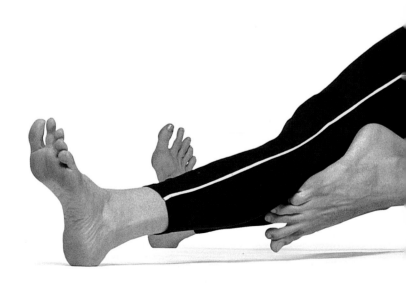

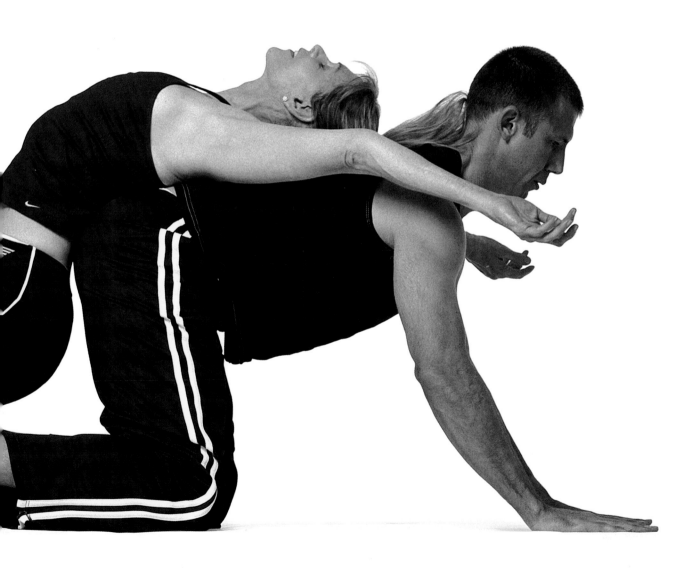

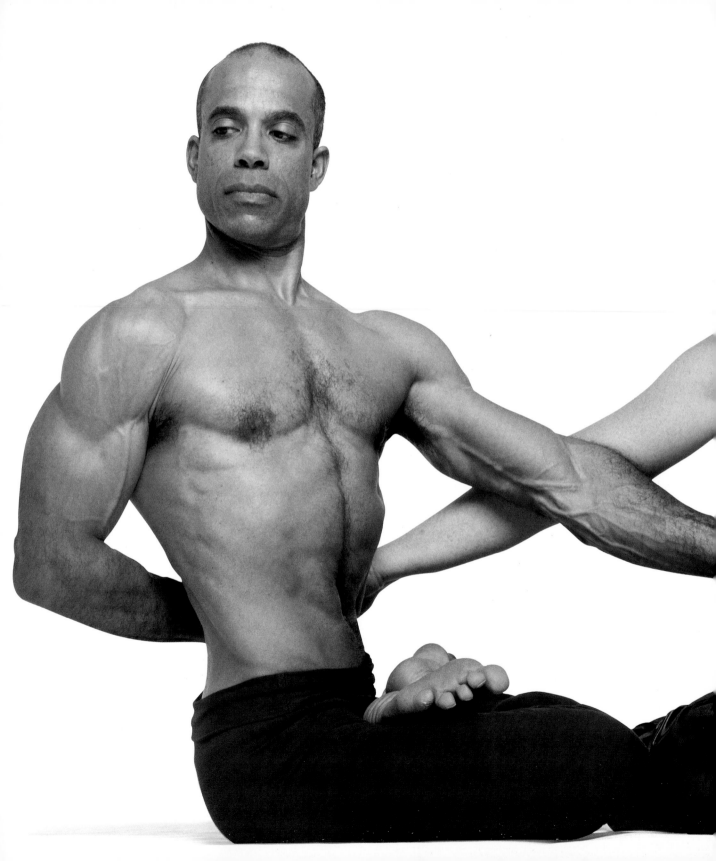

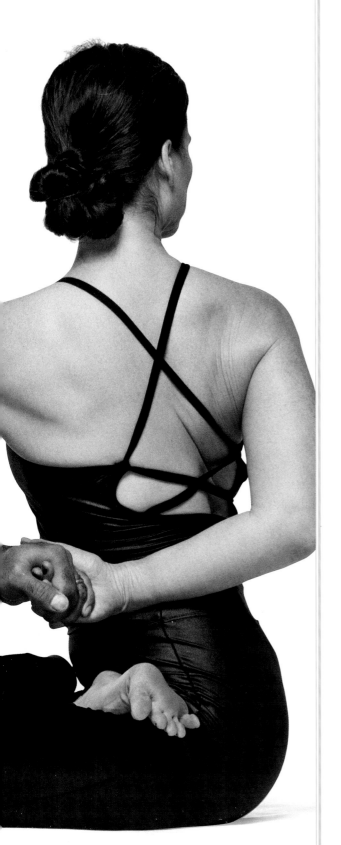

DOUBLE PRETZEL
JONATHAN & ANA

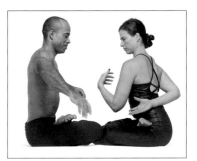

STEP 1 Jonathan and Ana sit cross-legged facing each other, knees touching.

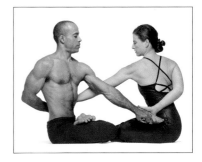

STEP 2 Both partners reach their right hands behind their backs and reach diagonally across the body with the left hand to clasp their partner's right hand.

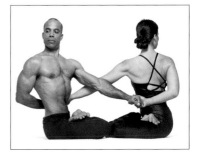

STEP 3 Turning away from each other, they twist, pulling gently with their right hands to increase the twist. Lifting on the inhalation and twisting deeper on the exhalation, they synchronize their breath and open deeply. They repeat on other side, placing left hands behind the back and reaching across with the right hand.

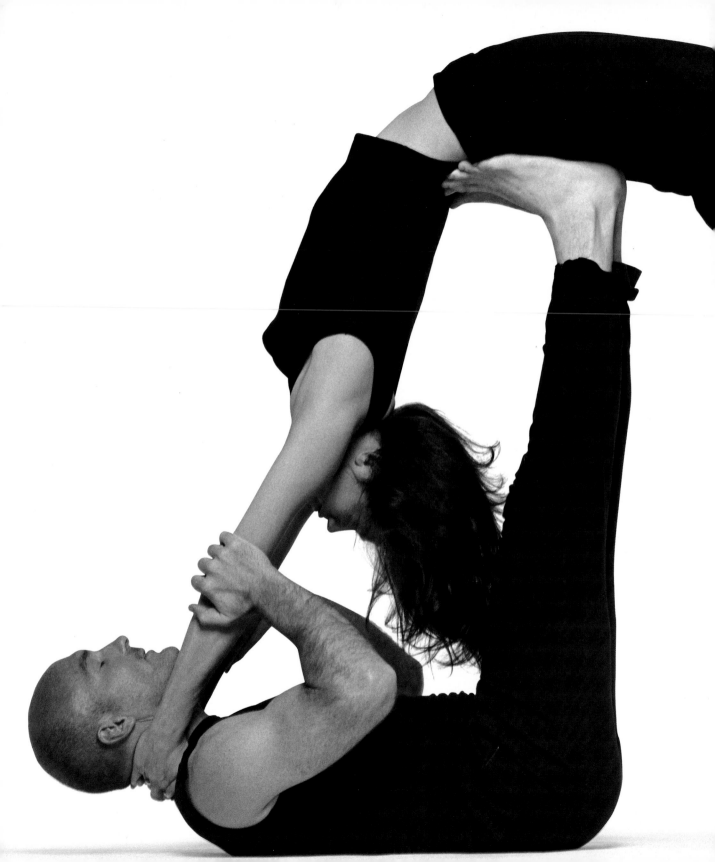

SHOOTING STAR

ELIZABETH & STEPHEN

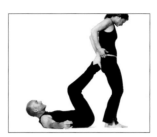

STEP 1 Elizabeth places Stephen's feet at a comfortable place on her lower back.

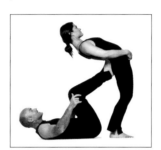

STEP 2 Elizabeth arches her back over Stephen's feet.

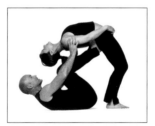

STEP 3 Stephen supports Elizabeth's backbend by holding and guiding her shoulders.

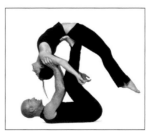

STEP 4 When Elizabeth is ready, Stephen presses his legs forward and straight to lift her off the ground.

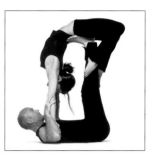

STEP 5 Elizabeth then hooks her feet around Stephen's legs. Reaching for Stephen's shoulders, she pulls herself into a deep stretch. Stephen assists by pulling Elizabeth's arms down.

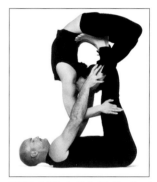

STEP 6 Elizabeth holds Stephen's legs to go even deeper into the stretch. Stephen guides her head to touch her feet.

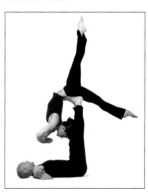

STEP 7 Elizabeth releases and elongates to transition to shooting star pose. Stephen balances her sacrum on his feet. Elizabeth scissors her legs and brings her hands together in prayer. Stephen holds her steady with firm legs, maintaining eye contact.

85

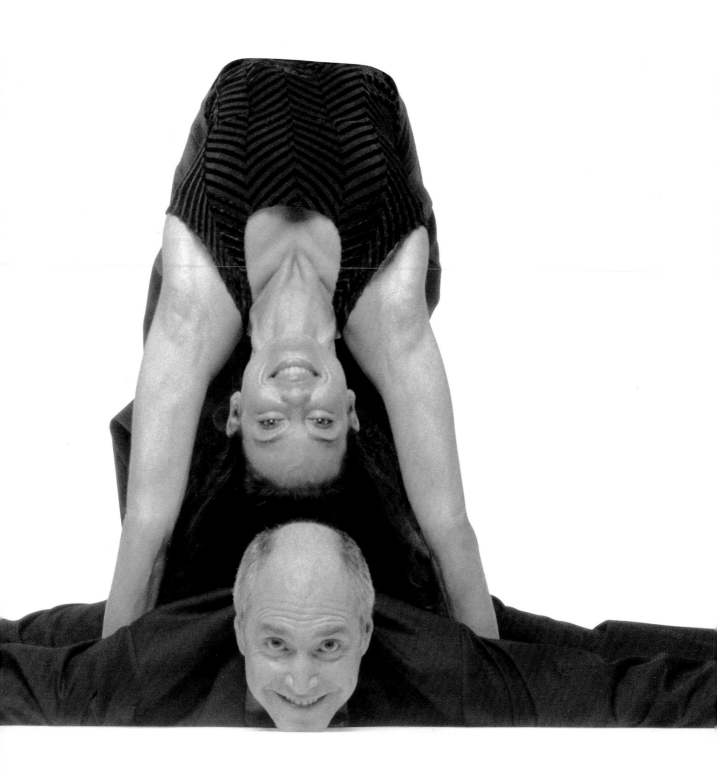

> *"Dissolve the boundaries that create separation while still remaining true to yourself. The flow of life is in the now."*
>
> —*Eckhart Tolle*

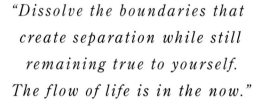

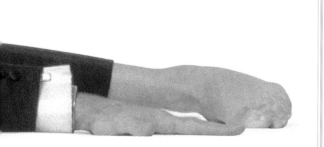

BALANCED "T"

JENNIFER & STEVE

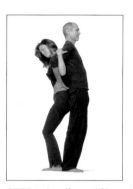

STEP 1 Jennifer and Steve stand back-to-back. Jennifer hooks Steve's arms over her shoulders like back-pack straps. She moves her buttocks into the small of his back.

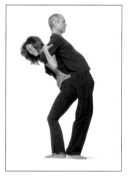

STEP 2 Jennifer bends forward, checking with Steve to make sure that she is supporting his back. Steve holds Jennifer's hips as he relaxes back over her.

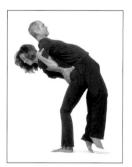

STEP 3 Jennifer continues to bend forward, lifting Steve's feet off the ground. She bends her knees to support his weight. He surrenders into the backbend.

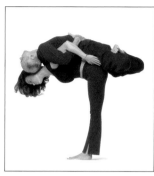

STEP 4 Steve brings his right leg into half lotus. Jennifer holds him steady on her back.

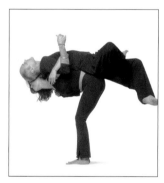

STEP 5 Steve brings his left leg up into full lotus. Jennifer hugs him to her back with her arms and elbows.

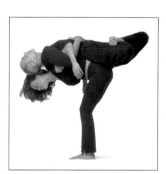

STEP 6 Jennifer straightens her legs as Steve lowers his knees, opening his groin.

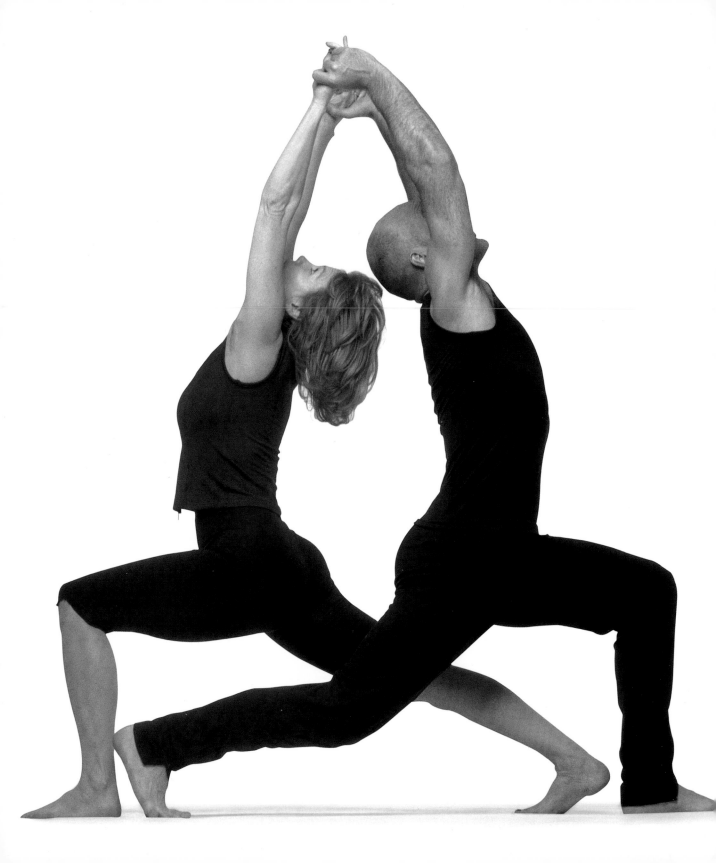

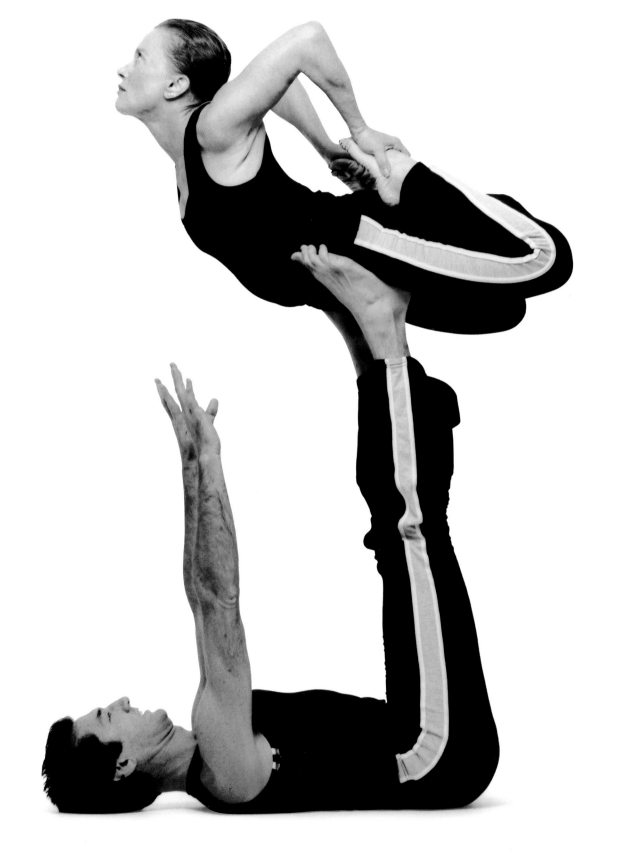

LOVE

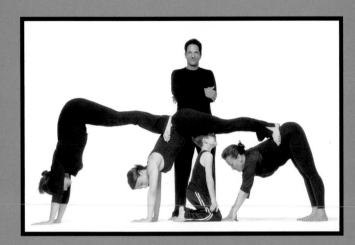

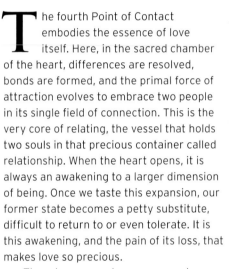

Qualities:

FORGIVENESS
COMPASSION
ACCEPTANCE

Gift:

INTIMACY

Challenge:

VULNERABILITY

The fourth Point of Contact embodies the essence of love itself. Here, in the sacred chamber of the heart, differences are resolved, bonds are formed, and the primal force of attraction evolves to embrace two people in its single field of connection. This is the very core of relating, the vessel that holds two souls in that precious container called relationship. When the heart opens, it is always an awakening to a larger dimension of being. Once we taste this expansion, our former state becomes a petty substitute, difficult to return to or even tolerate. It is this awakening, and the pain of its loss, that makes love so precious.

Though we crave love, we cannot use our will to make it happen. We can only surrender to the mystery of it and face the inevitable vulnerability that falling in love requires.

But how do you avoid those unconscious little things that diminish love—those careless words or acts that create distance or cause the heart to shut down? How do you remain true to yourself while entering more deeply into relationship with another? And how do you protect love from the stresses of daily life, keeping the spark strong year after year? These are the questions asked in any relationship.

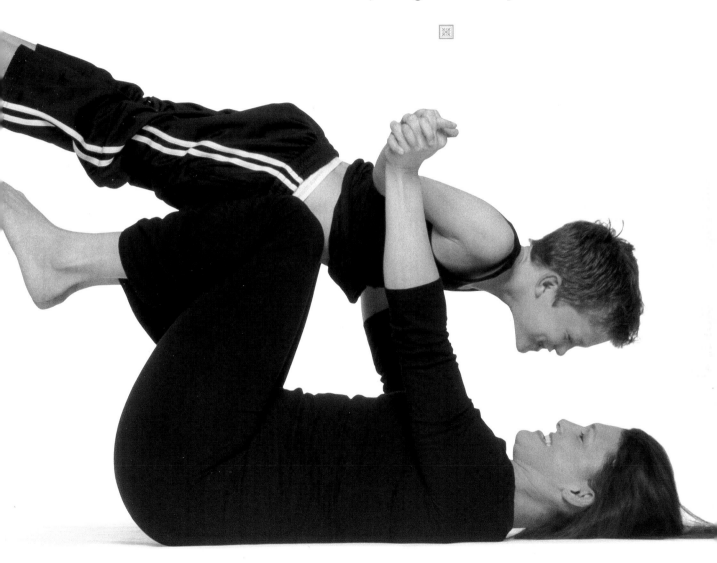

"Though we crave love, we cannot use our will to make it happen. We can only surrender to the mystery of it and face the inevitable vulnerability that falling in love requires."

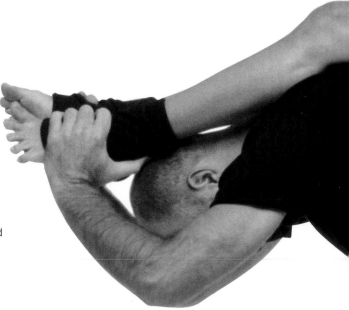

Our fourth Point of Contact occurs at the literal heart of the chakra system, with three chakras above and three below: it is the center, the fulcrum. To keep your relationship growing in the field of love, you must find balance, both within yourself and with your partner. This means balance between self and other, honoring both equally, neither one sacrificed for the other. Here you seek balance between giving and receiving, initiating and following. This center represents integration of body and mind, matter and spirit, inner and outer, activity and rest. It asks that we come into acceptance of ourselves and of another just as we are, with compassion and understanding.

We often think of love as a noun—something that we want to get, to own, to have—but it is most profoundly a verb. Love is something we do—it is an act of giving, of receiving someone else into your essential being, of making yourself open and vulnerable. Love is an act of commitment, of trust and understanding. Love arises from pleasure: it is kept intact through commitment and communication and nurtured by vision. It is the universal force that dissolves boundaries and leads to union.

We court love by loving, by engaging in a constant attitude of kindness, compassion, and forgiveness. We court love by making contact with the deep soul within ourselves and within another. We court love by seeing the divine Beloved in the face of the other and recognizing that face as a mirror of ourselves.

Love is an experience that takes place in the eternal present, as a state of being. It is an opportunity that exists in each precious moment. It is thwarted by resentment, bitterness, and holding on to the past. Forgiveness opens the heart and frees it from the past so you can be fully open to the possibilities of the present.

And finally, love's grace is most profoundly expressed through compassion and empathy. Compassion means to feel with someone, not that you have to fix what's wrong; in fact, often you can't. It just means that you can relate to your partner's struggle, suffering, or situation. A little compassion goes a long way toward encouraging the self within to come out and play. Only through acceptance, kindness, forgiveness, and compassion does the lotus of heart truly flower into the fullness of love.

The absence of love—its withdrawal or loss—brings grief. It feels like betrayal and closes down the heart, shutting down relationship. As you open your heart through some of these poses, old grief may surface and pour through. Open deeply to your grief, allowing your partner to simply meet it with compassion and empathy. Breathe into it and let its waves move through your body, up and out, releasing these deep pockets of emotion.

When the wells of grief are finally released, the lotus of the heart flowers once again. The breath expands, the eyes brighten, and the clouds part, revealing the radiant sun. To radiate from the heart is to shine forth from the center, whole and complete, and meet another in that radiance.

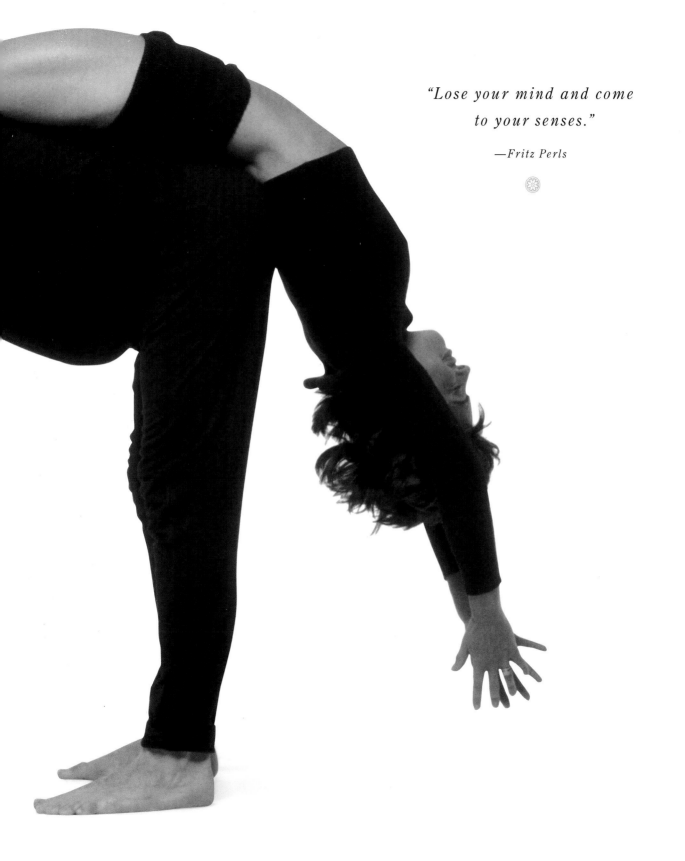

"*Lose your mind and come
to your senses.*"

—*Fritz Perls*

GUIDELINES FOR
LOVE
IN PRACTICE

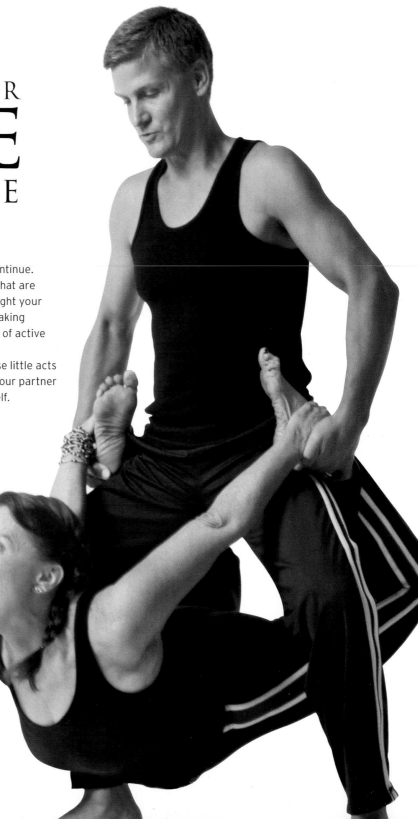

Love, like anything, must be nourished to continue. It thrives on kindness and consideration. What are the little acts you can do to surprise or delight your partner? What are the things that show you are taking him or her into consideration? What are the ways of active loving, of showing you truly care?

To invite love into your practice, embody those little acts of caring and tenderness. Show appreciation to your partner for the little things he or she does. Extend yourself.

1. **WORK WITH THE BREATH** since the element of the heart chakra is air. Breathing is an essential part of any yoga practice. In Contact, however, you must not only open your own breath, but also coordinate your breath with another to bring deeper contact and alignment.

2. **MELT INTO EACH OTHER.** Feel yourself soften, letting go of resistance to whatever contact you are making. Let yourself be fully present to meeting and being met. When two people embody this concept, they neither invade each other nor retreat from each other. They simply meet, consciously and creatively. Once you have entered fully into a pose, tune into the core energy running through your own center. Then move your attention slowly out from the core to the places where your two bodies are touching. Simply feel where they meet and slowly allow that frontier of flesh to expand.

3. **ALLOW YOUR BODY TO FORM AN OFFERING OF LOVE AND ACCEPTANCE.** Imagine your energy body has wings that caress your partner in tenderness, moving out from the muscles in your back, the bones of your sacrum, or the strength of your legs. As your partner expands toward you, accept each extension with gratitude and grace.

4. **INVITE YOUR PARTNER TO MEET YOU.** If he or she is less flexible than you are, you may have to stretch a little farther. And if your partner feels less than fully present at any time, you may have to resist overextending, instead holding your edge and encouraging your partner to come forward and meet you. Tell him where he can extend, reach, press, or move to meet you better. When he really connects, let him know, and then focus and deepen the experience at the frontiers of your meeting.

5. **EMBODY A SENSE OF EMPATHY TOWARD YOUR PARTNER.** Feel into her body as if it were your own. Find ways to communicate that empathy through your movements. Be patient and gentle, but encouraging.

6. **TREAT EACH CONTACT POSE LIKE AN EMBRACE.** Expand your consciousness into the contact the way you would embrace a loved one you haven't seen in a while. Embrace your differences as well—differences of height, flexibility, or strength—and use them to enhance the pose. Always find a way to work the pose to its fullest potential for contact.

*"One learns through the heart,
not the eyes or the intellect."*

—*Mark Twain*

BREATHING
EXERCISE

Before beginning a pose, take a moment to align your energies by breathing together. Whether standing face-to-face, sitting back-to-back, or in any preparatory position, listen to the rhythm of each other's breaths. Breathe out as your partner breathes in, and in as he breathes out, allowing the breath to be a continuous circle of exchange between you. While moving into a pose or adjusting into your final position, you may lose this coordination of breath, but once you are fully in the pose, pause and then realign your breath once more.

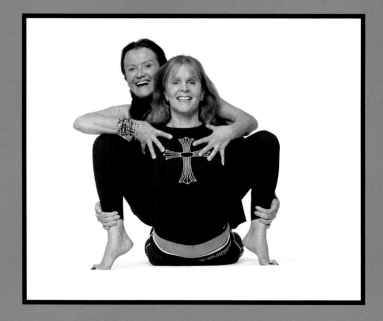

"If you are not in your body, you are not in your life. Breath is the tool that takes you there."

—*Tara Guber*

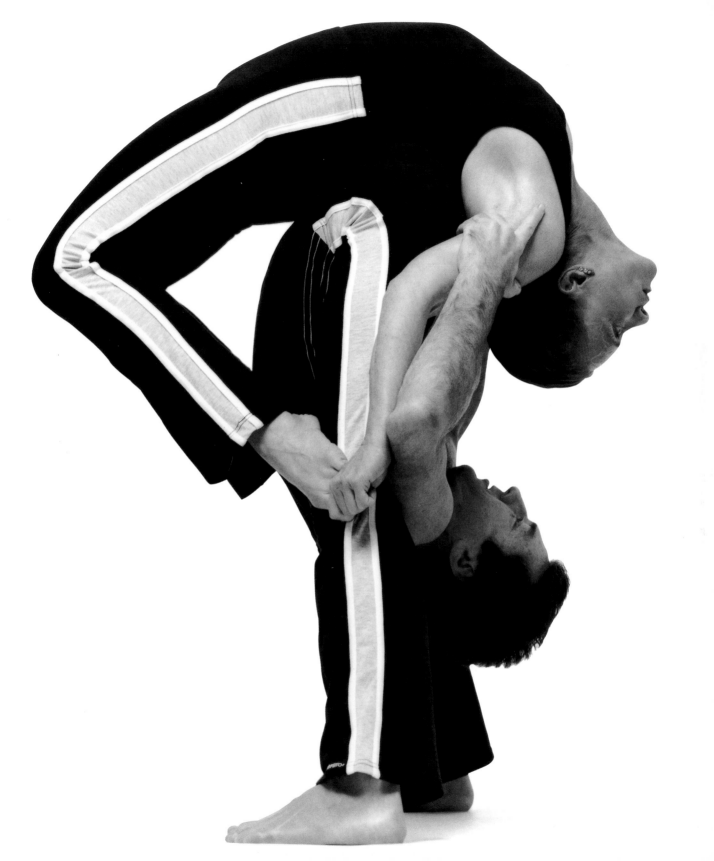

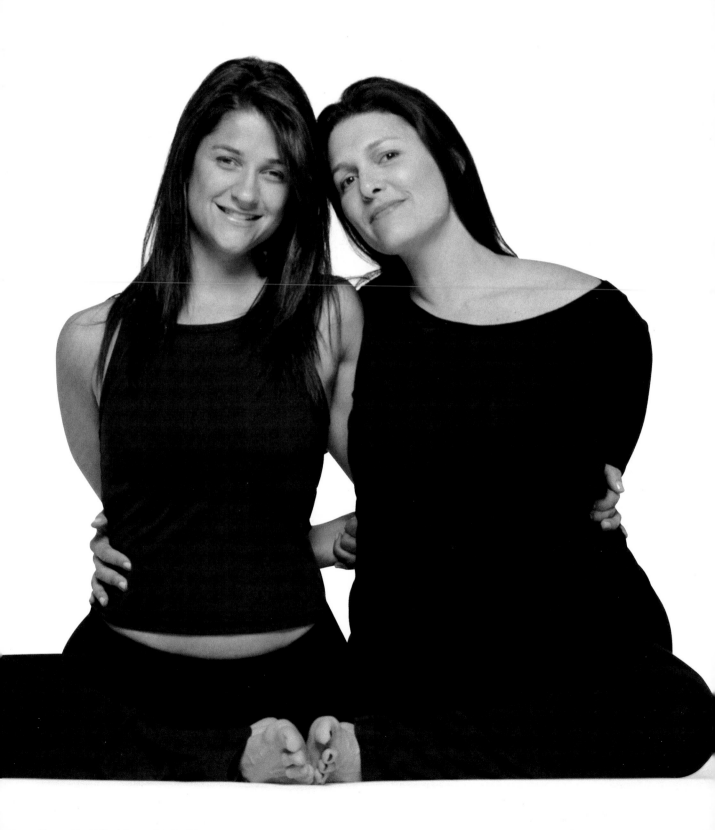

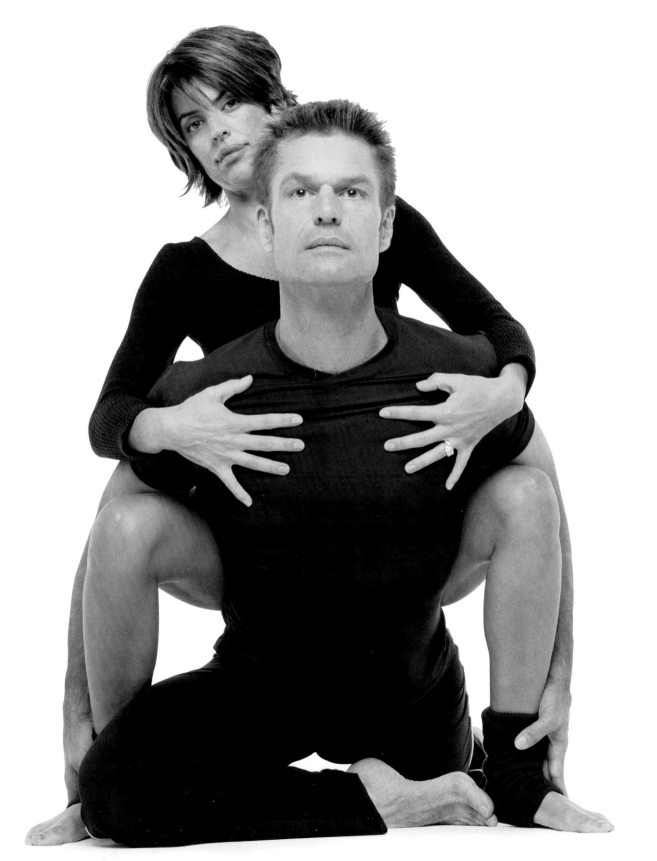

*"The only lasting beauty is the
beauty of the heart."*

—*Rumi*

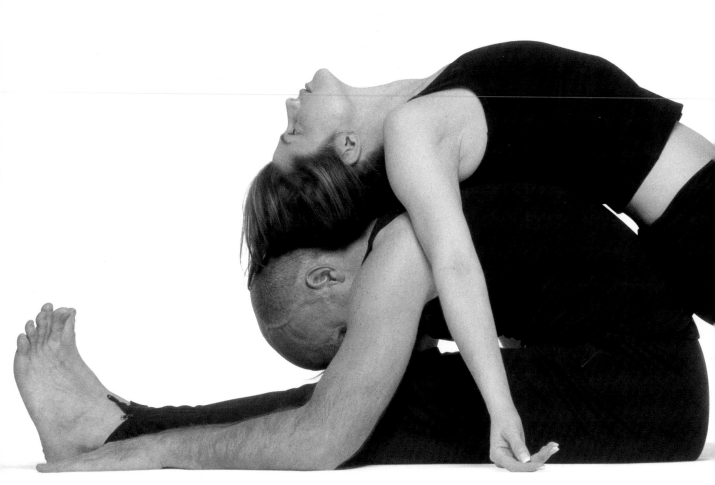

HEART & SHOULDER OPENER

STEPHEN & DAPHNE

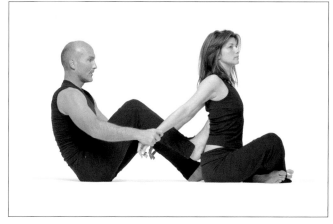

STEP 1 Stephen holds Daphne by the wrists as he massages her sacrum with his feet.

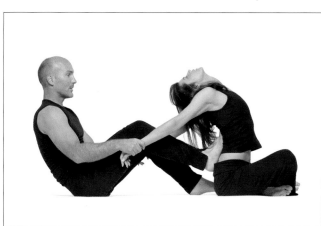

STEP 2 Continuing to massage her lower back, he begins to gently stretch her arms to open up her shoulders and then her heart.

UPPER-BODY STRETCH
TARA & DEVARSHI

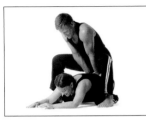

STEP 1 Tara rests her torso on her thighs, her knees open and feet together. Devarshi places his palms on Tara's sacrum and gently applies pressure back and down to open up her hips.

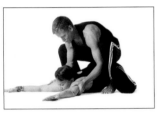

STEP 2 Devarshi places his hands above Tara's elbows and begins to stretch and elongate both sides of her body.

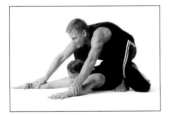

STEP 3 Devarshi continues to work his hands down Tara's arms, resulting in a gentle stretch of the upper body.

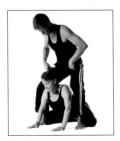

STEP 4 Tara places her hands on the floor and straightens her arms as she comes up to sitting. Devarshi begins to squat.

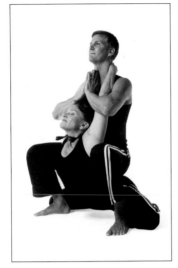

STEP 5 Devarshi helps Tara place her hands and, ideally, interlace her fingers behind his neck. Devarshi places his sitting bones on Tara's sacrum.

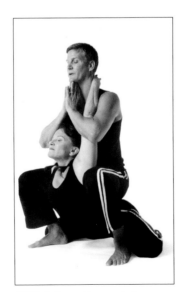

STEP 6 Devarshi supports Tara and allows his sitting bones to gently stretch her sacrum down and back as she surrenders to a fully openhearted backbend.

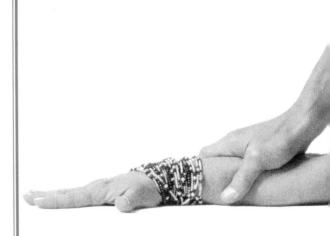

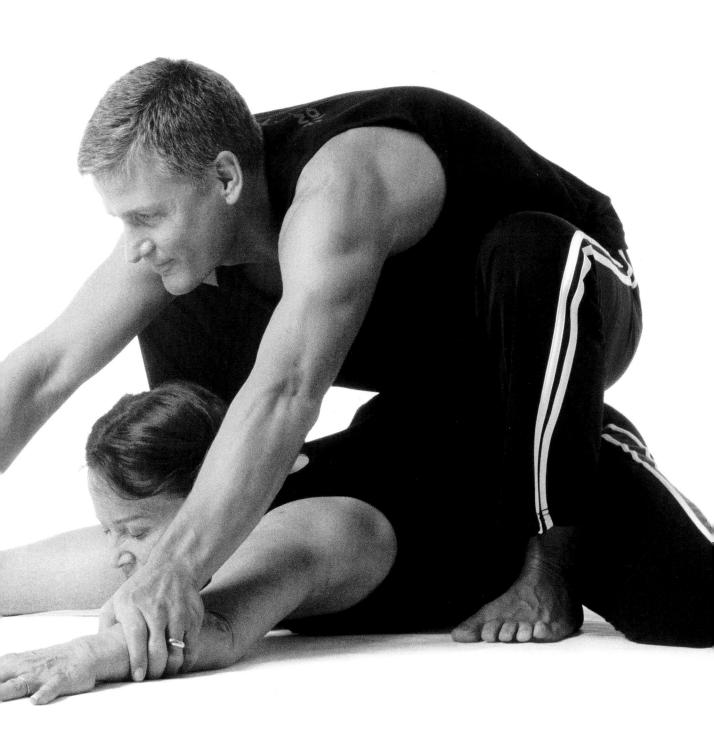

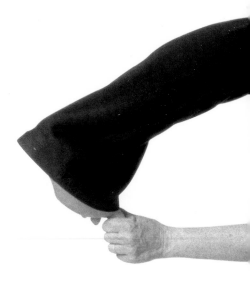

*"If you tell the truth you don't
have to remember anything."*

—*Mark Twain*

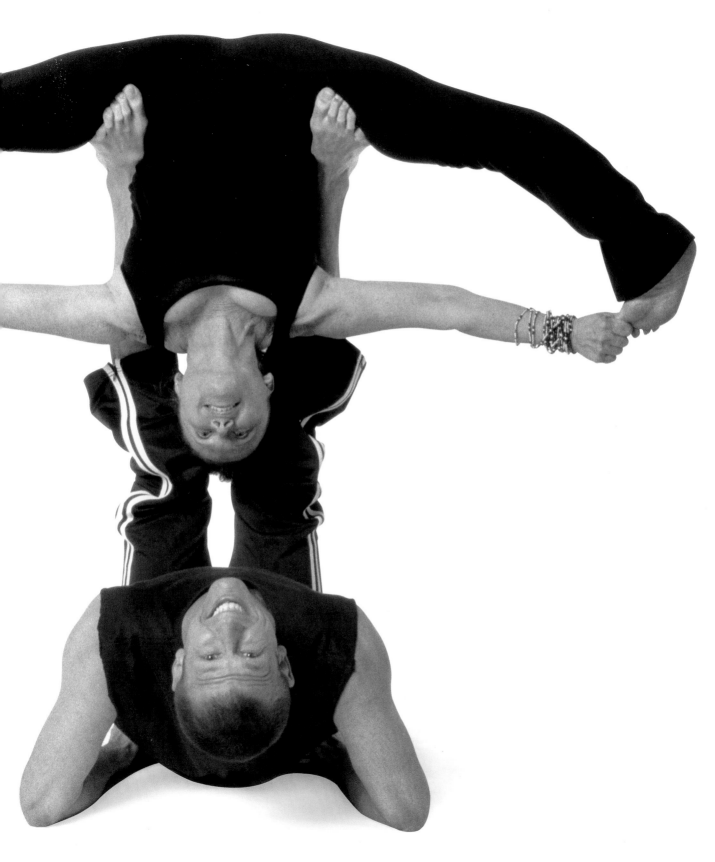

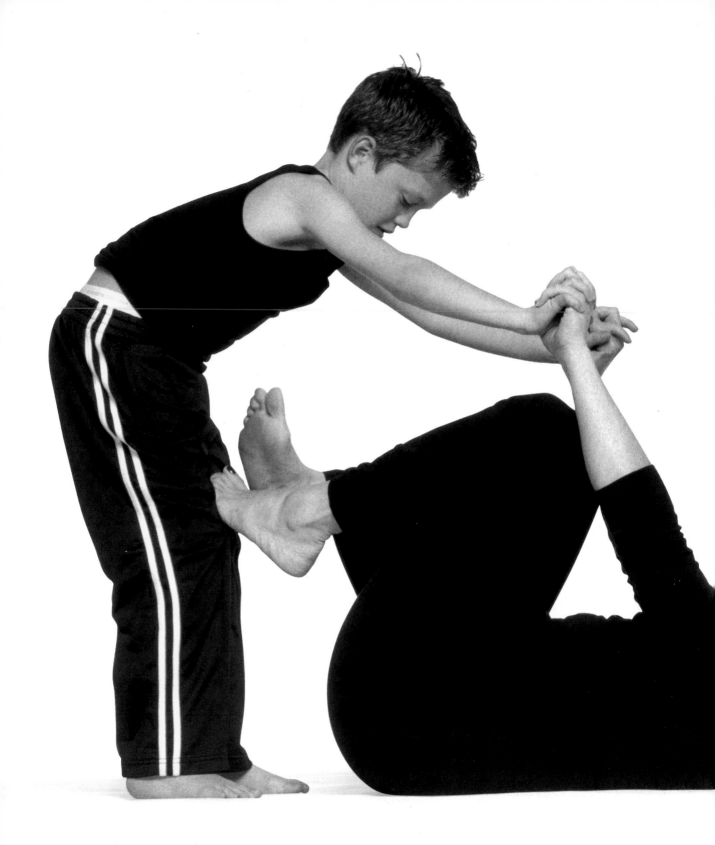

> *"It is only with the heart that one can see rightly; what is essential is invisible to the eye."*
>
> —*Antoine de Saint-Exupéry*

FLYING THRONE
JODI & JAXON

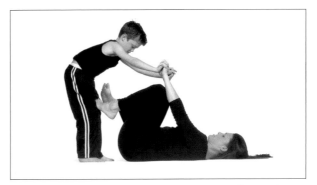

STEP 1 Jodi clasps hands with her brother Jaxon. Jodi moves her feet between his legs to rest under his buttocks.

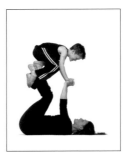

STEP 2 Jodi presses her legs forward and straight to lift Jaxon off the ground.

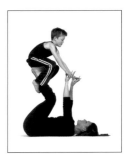

STEP 3 Jaxon engages his own core lower-torso strength to shift his weight back. He carefully releases Jodi's hands.

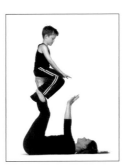

STEP 4 Jaxon sits up tall while maintaining eye contact. Jodi supports him, finding his relative alignment and balance. She maintains a strong and steady leg position.

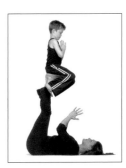

STEP 5 When they have found a consistent steady balance, Jodi fully straightens her legs. They both bring their hands to their hearts and share in light and love.

COMMUNICATION

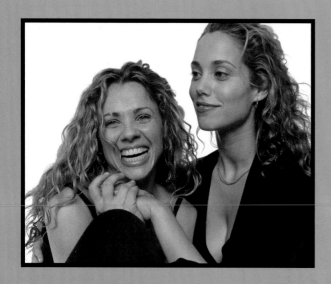

Qualities:

CONVERSATION
CONNECTION
HONESTY

Gift:

RAPPORT

Challenge:

DISTANCE

If love contains relationship, communication holds it together. It connects the pieces, mends the fragments when they break, and shapes the vessel to fit the partners involved. Without communication, there is no way to protect yourself or your partner, no way to express your appreciation or make your needs known. It takes communication to fulfill each of the other Points of Contact, just as it takes trust, passion, commitment, love, and vision to communicate. Communication is vital to this practice.

Why? Because Contact Yoga happens in the moment. It is not a preordained set of precise postures but a dynamic and continuous creative flow between two people, guided by constant communication. Communication guides the subtle streams of energy within you into the rivers of connection. It literally tells the rivers where to go: more here, less there, ooh that's great, just like that. Directing the flow makes the difference between an active and a passive practice.

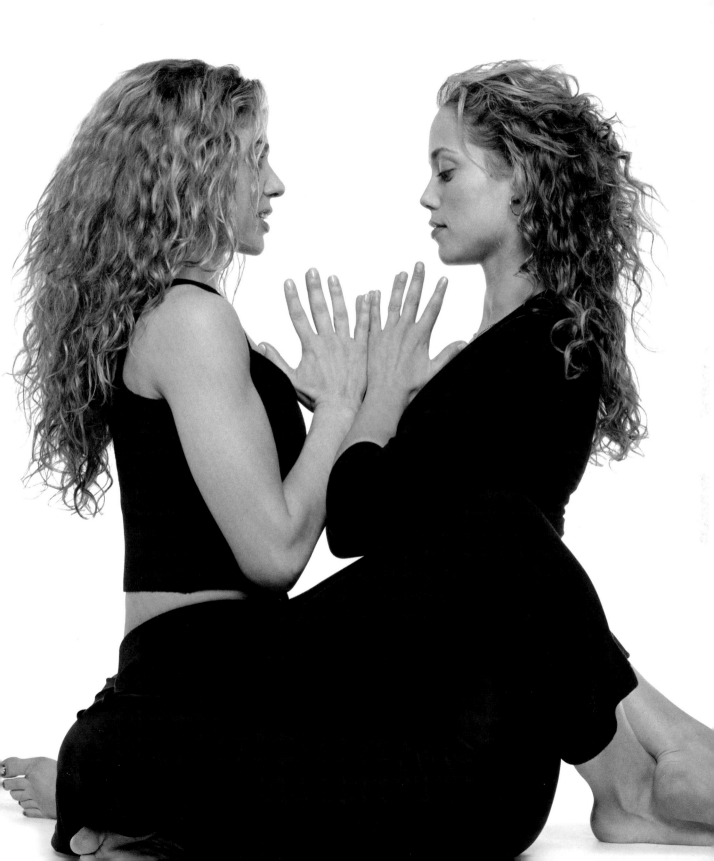

Without communication, there is no relationship. The flow between two people is blocked, and they remain isolated in their separate realities. They can't find their places of agreement or disagreement. They can't direct their energies. They relate to assumptions and projections instead of relating to each other. When this happens, you need to go back inside yourself to find your own truth and bring it out. If this fifth Point of Contact is kept open, even difficult communications can lead to greater intimacy.

In Contact Yoga, there are many ways to communicate. Words, sounds, movements, gestures, breath—all flow together like lines of poetry, punctuated by grunts and laughter. When you find the areas of connection, you feel the harmony. When you get just the right place in a pose, you both feel it. At that moment, you might yell out, "Contact!"

Contact is a way that two people can speak the language of yoga together. For those with a solitary practice, this is a profound opening. Like any language, it deepens and becomes more meaningful when you can speak it with someone else.

The more fluently your body speaks the vocabulary of *asanas*,

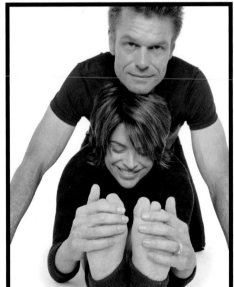

or yoga postures, the more deeply you can converse in this practice. When two people have a solid knowledge of their own bodies and have both strength and flexibility, honed from years of regular yoga practice, the Contact conversation is eloquent. It flows back and forth in intricate beauty. As beginners experience Contact, they begin to learn this language, and as they return to the mat for their own practice, their understanding of Contact increases.

Communication is where the inside comes out; this is an important barrier to cross. How often have you sensed something in your partner's mood but didn't know what it was really about? You can tune into the subtle nuances of your partner's body language, but it's all guesswork unless he tells you what's going on. Only by sharing this deep interior do we create the connection from the inner world that really brings intimacy. When the insides connect through communication and the outsides connect through Contact, you have an amazing combination that creates profound rapport.

Not all communication leads directly to intimacy, however. Sometimes communication creates distance, fear, or worry. Sometimes honesty feels dangerous, coming through like a knife or breaking down completely. Then you can move to other forms of communication—through the body, breath, sounds, or gestures. Use any of the other Points of Contact to rebuild your connection, starting with the base of trust.

And what do we most need to communicate? Our own truth, whatever that may be. In yoga philosophy, truth is described by the word *satya*, which simply means "what is." Outside of our personal value system, the truth is neither good nor bad, but just the way things happen to be. We can fight it and resist, or we can find ways to relate to it. When we embrace communication with an open mind and heart, we make contact.

When shared in relationship, truth tunes the instruments so they can play together. How can this be done if only one of you makes a sound? And how can you play together if there is no attunement? No attunement, no attainment; it's as simple as that.

When two people are well tuned to each other and the communication channels are open, there is the possibility of harmony. Each person can then be true to themselves, true to their word, and true to their partner. This harmony is essential for the deep union that is the ultimate goal of yoga.

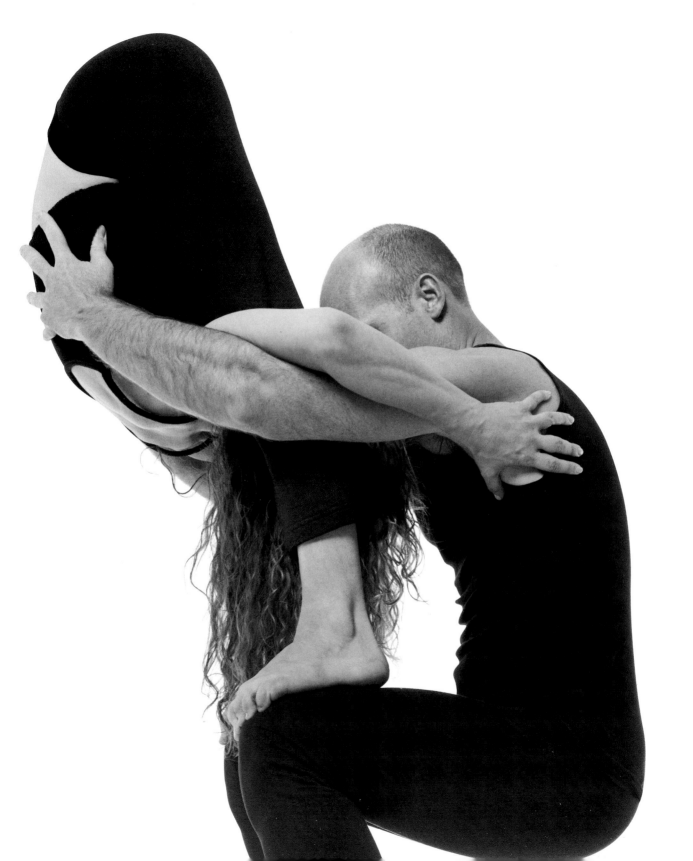

GUIDELINES FOR
COMMUNICATION
IN PRACTICE

So many of us find it hard to ask for what we want: a softer touch, a stronger presence, more honest communication, a moment of being heard or understood. And there are so many levels involved in communication. You can speak with your eyes, your body movements, your breath, your touch. The most obvious communication is with words, but if your body is arched over mine, there is also the communication of the tension you hold in your muscles and the energetic presence that's present or missing in your body. These subtle signals go on all the time beneath our awareness, but in Contact, we seek to make them conscious.

Learn to listen with all your senses. Even before words are spoken, listen to your partner's body language to see if she is ready and present. Listen for the places that are blocked or hesitant, the places that need to stretch and release.

Look for subtle movements and facial expressions, especially in the eyes, to see if there is fear or insecurity. You can listen to the breath to better synchronize with your partner or to know when she is holding back. These things can then be brought into verbal communication—"slow down," "move a little this way," "feel my support," "relax your breath." This is the refinement that allows you to really align your energy with another.

❧ ❧ ❧ ❧ ❧

1. **LEARN YOUR PARTNER'S LANGUAGE.** He or she may have a different way of moving or speaking than you. As you learn each other's language, begin to create a common language for Contact. Words and phrases will spontaneously arise that describe certain feelings. Develop fluency in all levels of communication as well as your own language of intimacy. This will do wonders to build trust.

2. **LISTEN, REFLECT, AND RESPOND.** Take a moment of silence before you speak. Mirror your partner's words or body language. Stay in the moment; this is critical. Let your partner know that she is heard and understood before moving on.

3. **COMMUNICATE WHAT YOU WANT AND NEED DIRECTLY AND SIMPLY:** your partner will not know how to give it to you unless you speak up. Take the guesswork out of your practice. Say no immediately to anything that doesn't feel right. Don't be afraid to ask—it's far better than assuming. "Is it OK like that?" "Do you want more here?" "Are you ready for this?"

4. **USE YOUR WORDS TO SHAPE REALITY, NOT TO NEGATE IT.** Be precise; stay positive. You can say, "I like it when you do that," rather than "Don't do it that way." Use your words to direct, not to criticize or limit your partner's energy.

5. **MAKE LOTS OF NOISE.** Don't be afraid to groan. Don't hold back. Sound moves energy through and releases pain and tension from your body.

6. **ONCE YOU'VE PRACTICED FOR A WHILE,** spend a session without words, just communicating through your bodies. Or, in your relationship, spend a day in silence together. Or simply spend a day with a determined commitment to avoid criticizing. For many couples, that change alone makes a big difference.

7. **LISTEN TO AND TRUST YOUR BODY.** The body doesn't lie. By having a practice that involves the body and reveals the ways your body connects, resonates, and speaks, core truths are revealed. Stay in communication with your body's needs, limitations, expansions, and fears. Communicate these inner nuances as best you can.

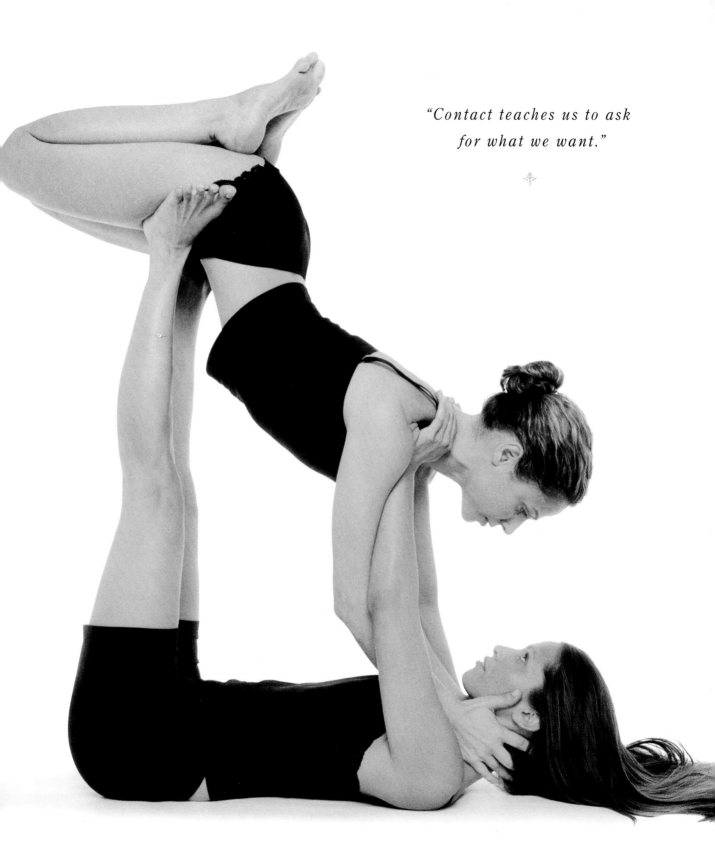

*"Contact teaches us to ask
for what we want."*

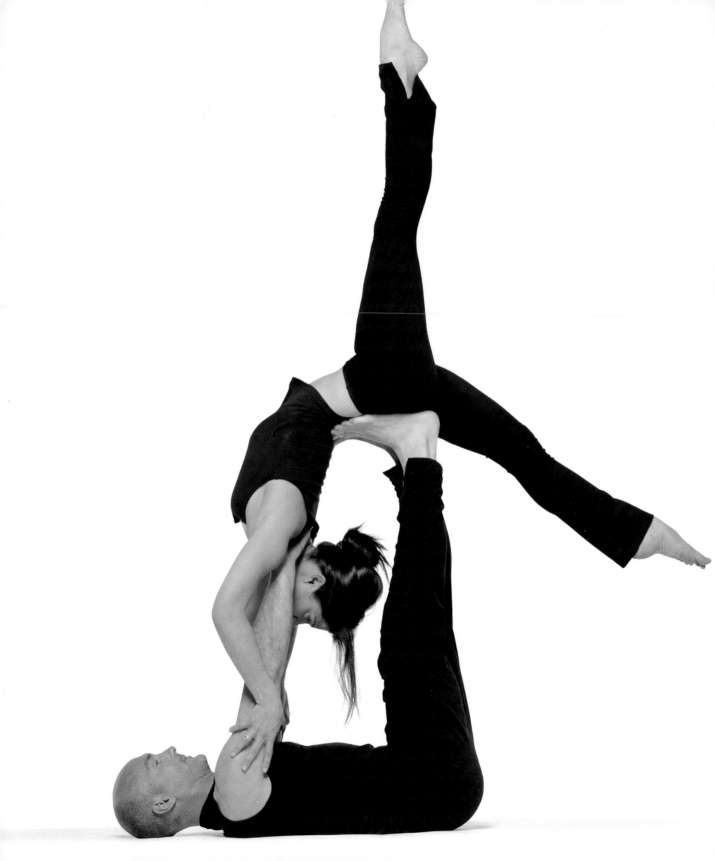

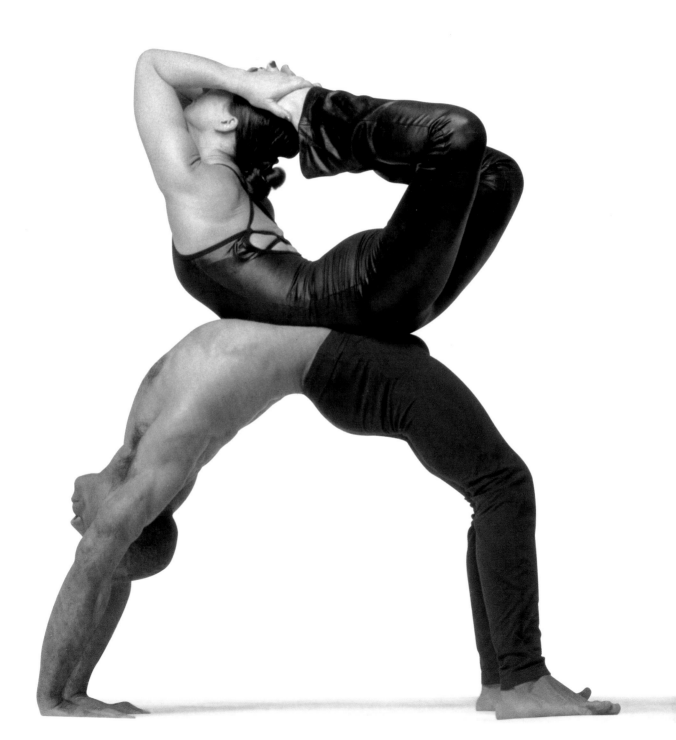

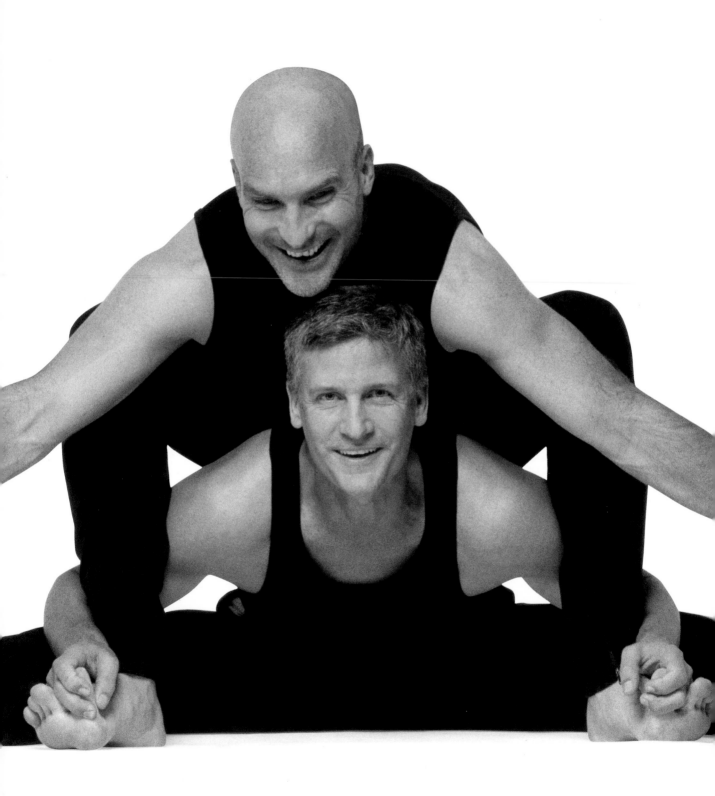

BEHIND-THE-BACK BOAT POSE

DEVARSHI & STEPHEN

"Our lives improve only when we take chances—and the first and most difficult risk we can take is to be honest with ourselves."

—Walter Anderson

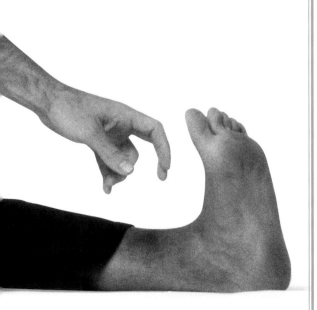

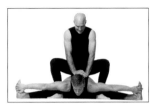

STEP 1 Devarshi starts in a wide-legged forward fold. Stephen places his feet along Devarshi's torso and sits gently on Devarshi's sacrum. Stephen lengthens Devarshi's sacrum and back with his sitting bones while stretching Devarshi's spine forward and down with his hands. They move slowly and communicate continually as they explore sensation and breath.

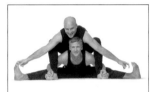

STEP 2 Stephen moves into a forward squat by reaching over Devarshi's shoulders. Devarshi hooks Stephen's toes to leverage himself forward for a groin stretch.

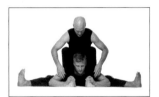

STEP 3 Stephen hooks his knees over Devarshi's shoulders. Devarshi stretches and massages Stephen's ankles and feet.

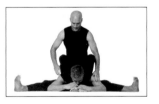

STEP 4 Devarshi grips Stephen's ankles and pulls them together as they prepare to transition into a strength and balance pose.

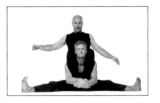

STEP 5 Stephen sits up and leans back as Devarshi holds his legs firmly in place. They move deeply into each other through breath, awareness, and communication.

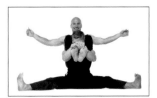

STEP 6 Devarshi sits up as Stephen leans back even further into the pose.

FLYING BUG
ON A BRIDGE
ANA & JONATHAN

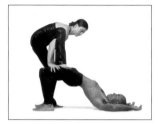

STEP 1 Jonathan lies down and lifts his hips up into a very solid bridge pose.

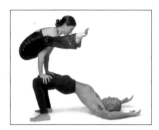

STEP 4 Ana lifts her other leg.

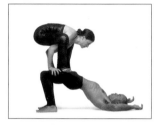

STEP 2 Ana places one hand and one foot on each of his thighs, elbows slightly bent.

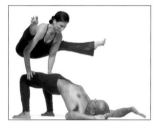

STEP 5 Looking with focus into each other's eyes, Jonathan and Ana go for it, stretching fully into this amazing advanced pose.

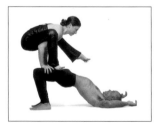

STEP 3 Maintaining eye contact and establishing trust, Ana lowers the backs of her thighs onto the shelf she has created with her arms, and begins to extend one leg.

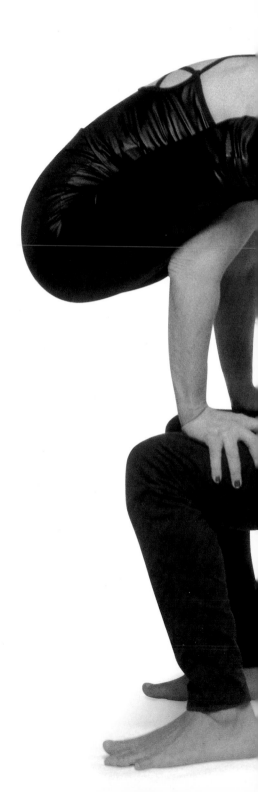

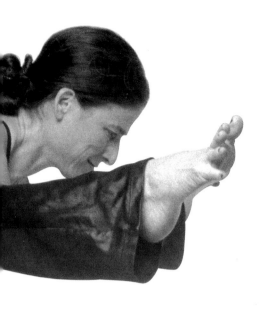

"Good communication is as
stimulating as black coffee and
just as hard to sleep after."

—*Anne Morrow Lindbergh*, Gift from the Sea

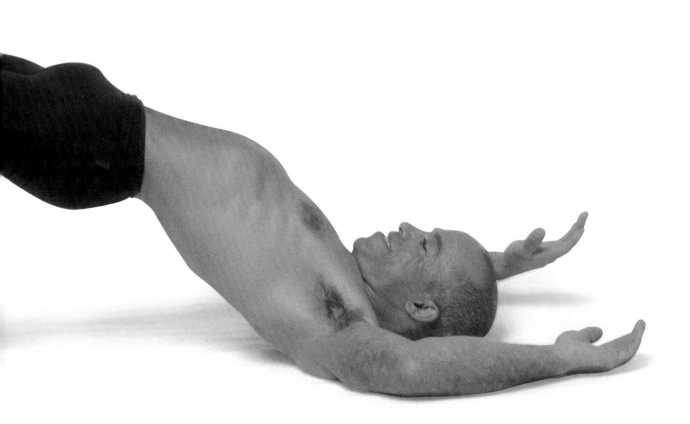

VISION

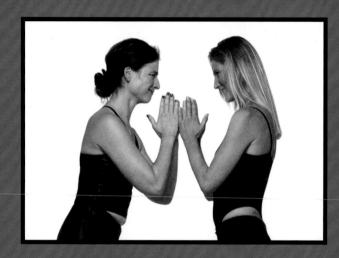

Qualities:

INTUITION
FOCUS
CREATIVITY

Gift:

CLARITY

Challenge:

ILLUSION

There's nothing like clarity in a relationship to make two people really shine together. You can see it when they walk down the street. There's a common rhythm to their steps, a light in their faces. It seems as if they communicate visually, confirmed by a mere look, a raise of the eyebrow, a gesture, or a smile.

Clarity has boldness and purpose to it, yet it has ease as well. With clarity, the struggle is resolved, either within yourself or between you and your partner. When it happens, you breathe a sigh of relief. At last you can let all of yourself go in one direction. What was previously caught up in searching or doubting can now relax and move forward. Clarity opens the way for a common vision.

In relationship, clarity comes when two people share a common vision. It may result from speaking the truth and clearing the air. It may come from a feeling of resonance that puts both partners on the same wavelength. It may come from surrendering to trust and transcending resistance. Or it may emerge from agreeing to a commitment, resolving issues of struggle and direction.

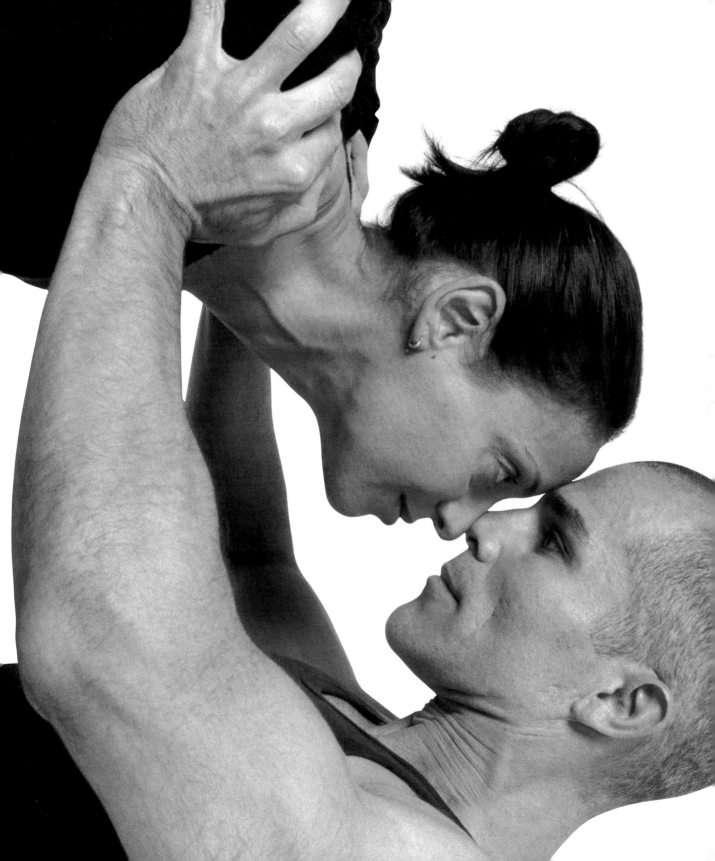

Clarity requires seeing and being seen clearly, essential aspects to feeling loved. It's something most of us long for and fear simultaneously. We want to be seen just as we are, without pretense, but that exposes the flaws as well as the beauty. Will we be accepted? Only when we no longer fear exposure will we make full and deep contact.

To see clearly, you have to really look beyond the usual projections, expectations, and filters that stand between yourself and others. You must release your preconceived notions and see things without distortion. And when you do, you may see the divine presence of your partner shining out through his eyes, hiding behind the fear and insecurities. This genuine insight into the eternal presence within calls that presence forth and lets it shine.

Only when you share this insight with your partner can you build a common vision. This inspirational pull from the future informs your direction, your actions, and your decisions here and now. It compels the relationship forward with purpose, helping it transcend the minor difficulties we all face. As it is something to work toward, vision makes it more likely that your relationship will have a future. It gives you something to aspire to, something bigger than your own needs. When achieved, your vision gives a glow of accomplishment that feeds the relationship with satisfaction.

The sixth Point of Contact opens when there is a common vision. This takes the relationship beyond desire for each other and into a higher purpose. The vision can be large or small, immediate to your daily circumstances or an offering to the world. For some, this vision may be raising their children, running a business together, supporting each other's growth, or finding a new balance between masculine and feminine.

If the vision does not extend beyond the sight of your beloved, the relationship will be limited. But when a higher purpose is served, that higher purpose informs the relationship in turn.

Vision arises out of the archetypal framework of the persons involved. What are your roles in the relationship? How and why did you pick those roles? What are you trying to accomplish in your own life, and how does relationship play into that? How do your roles and those of your partner fit together to form a common theme?

The challenge of this Point is to see through illusion. Our perceptions are so often filtered through our interpretations, our inner "movie" of how something should look, that we fail to see how it is. We project, deny, fabricate, imagine, and fantasize to reinforce the "reality" of our "movie." Whenever we do any of these, we pull ourselves out of contact. This yoga is not a virtual practice, but intensely real and present. Piercing through illusion is a liberating experience.

Vision arises out of our passion and is enacted through commitment, nourished through love, and expanded through communication. As we unite in vision, we become ready to take the final step into grace and experience union.

"You are here to enable the divine purpose of the universe to unfold. That is how important you are."

—*Eckhart Tolle*

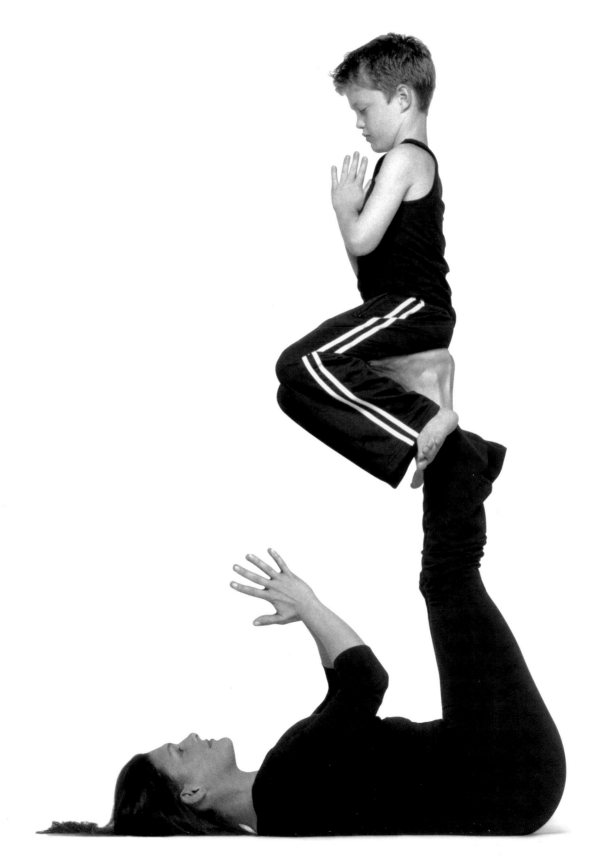

GUIDELINES FOR
VISION
IN PRACTICE

Whenever you practice Contact, take a moment to create a common vision for your practice that day. It might be to soothe a previous disagreement, find new inspiration, or keep a commitment. You might dedicate your practice to world peace or simply to inner peace, or seek healing in your back or in your heart.

Sometimes, one person has a vision for the day and needs to lead the other. Can you let yourself surrender to what your partner has in mind and really embrace her vision? On another day, can you enroll your partner in your own vision and lead the way? Can you move from holding separate visions to finding a common vision?

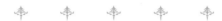

1. **SEEK TO SEE EYE-TO-EYE WITH YOUR PARTNER—LITERALLY.** This occurs in any pose that brings you face-to-face. Lock your gazes together in total focus and concentration. Stop. Breathe. Relax and open to the presence in front of you. Say hello with your eyes. Gazing into your partner's eyes, you can really see what's going on, see when fear or pleasure are present. This invites the spirit to show up, as well as the body. It helps you stay focused and enables trust to form.

2. **DON'T BE AFRAID TO BE SEEN.** Allow yourself to come out of hiding and let your eyes be windows to the soul. Try to communicate your fears, your excitement, and your love through your eyes. Relax your face and let your emotions show. Take a risk; reach beyond your normal boundaries. Expose yourself.

3. **FIND THE BEAUTY IN YOUR POSES TOGETHER.** Feel that beauty from within as you move, entering the deepest experience of Contact.

4. **REFLECT BEAUTY BACK TO YOUR PARTNER.** Express what you see. Tell him how strong his legs look when he's holding you. Tell her that her face is radiant. Describe how her eyes shine, or how secure you feel in his arms.

5. **BEGIN WITH THE END IN MIND.** Make each pose a work of art, an expression of vision, and an offering to spirit. Find the place in the pose that best lets the radiance of the energy body shine forth to your partner, as if you were making an offering of your body as art.

6. **IF YOU LOSE CONTACT WITH YOURSELF,** close your eyes and go back inside. Then slowly open them again, bringing forth what you find within. Let your inner witness see yourself and your partner at the same time.

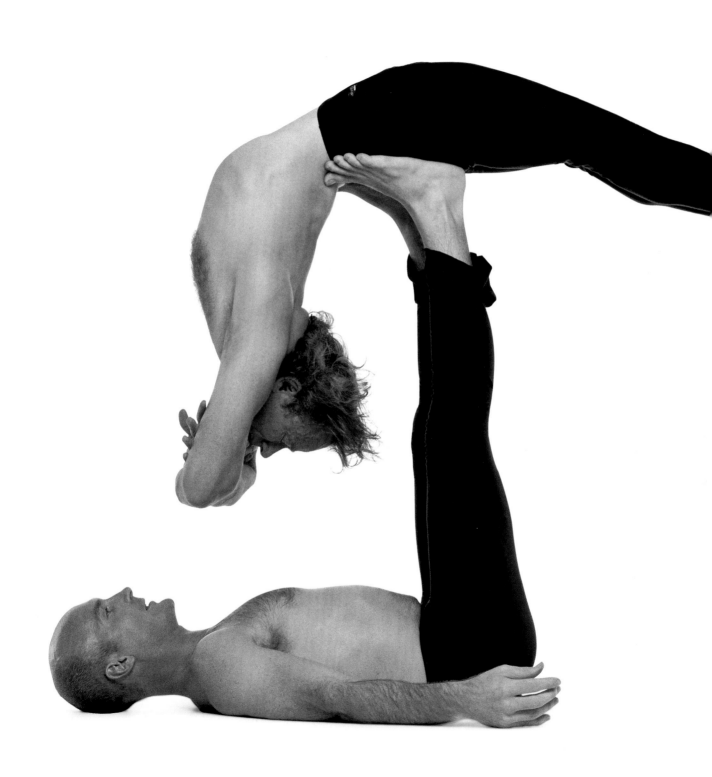

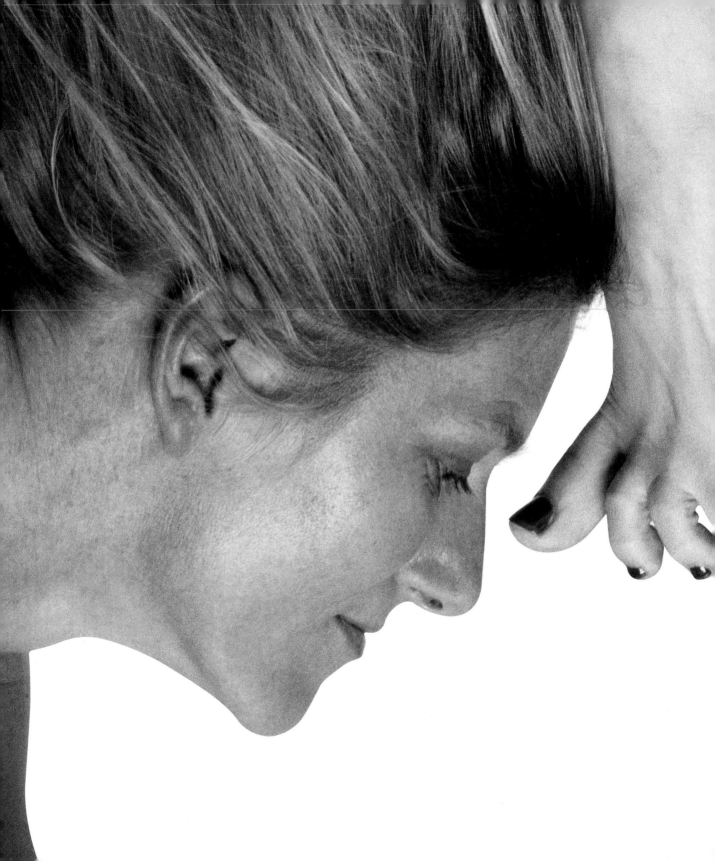

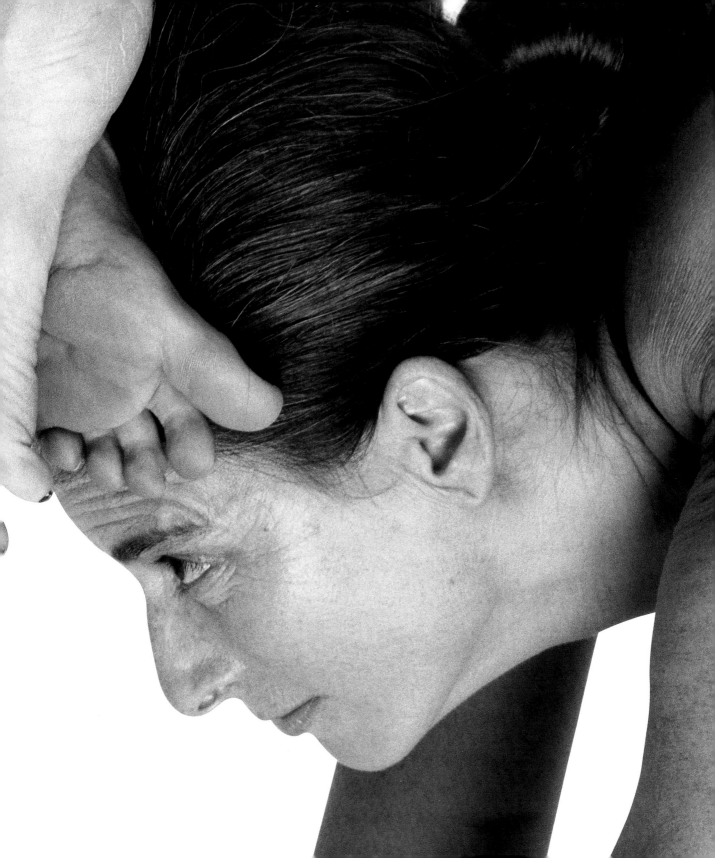

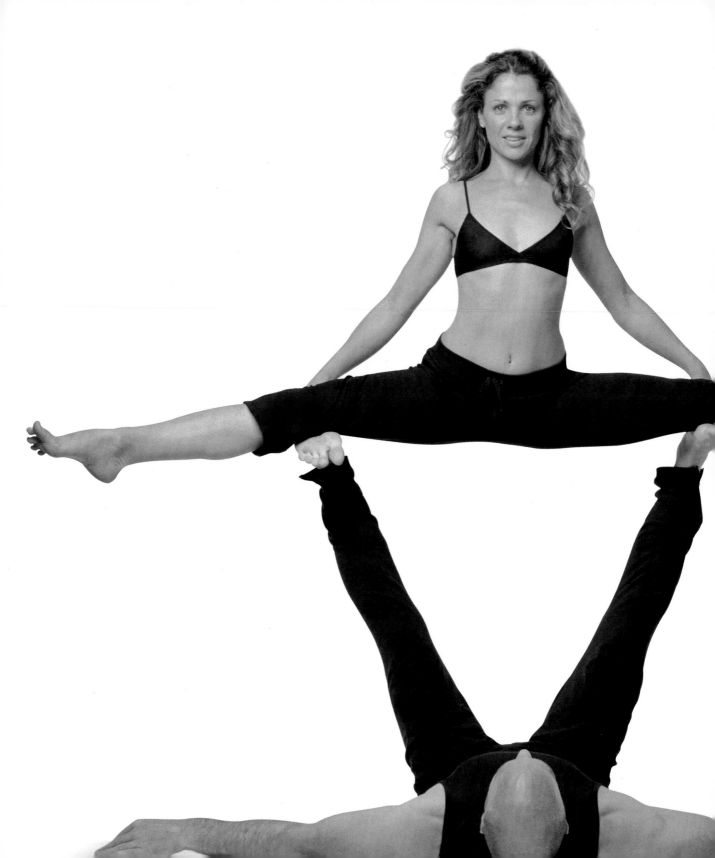

FLYING SPLITS

SEANE & STEPHEN

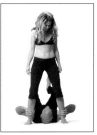

STEP 1 Seane stands with her feet on either side of Stephen's head. Stephen grips her ankles firmly.

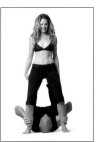

STEP 2 Stephen bends his knees and brings his feet up. Seane leans and reaches back to place them on her thighs.

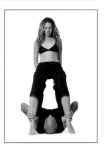

STEP 3 As Seane sits back onto his flexed feet, Stephen lifts her legs up to a sitting position.

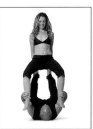

STEP 4 Stephen straightens his legs and widens his feet as Seane establishes her balance in a wide-legged position.

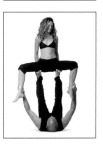

STEP 5 Stephen spreads his feet wider to support Seane in extending her legs straight.

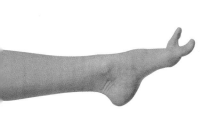

"Imagination is more important than knowledge."

—*Albert Einstein*

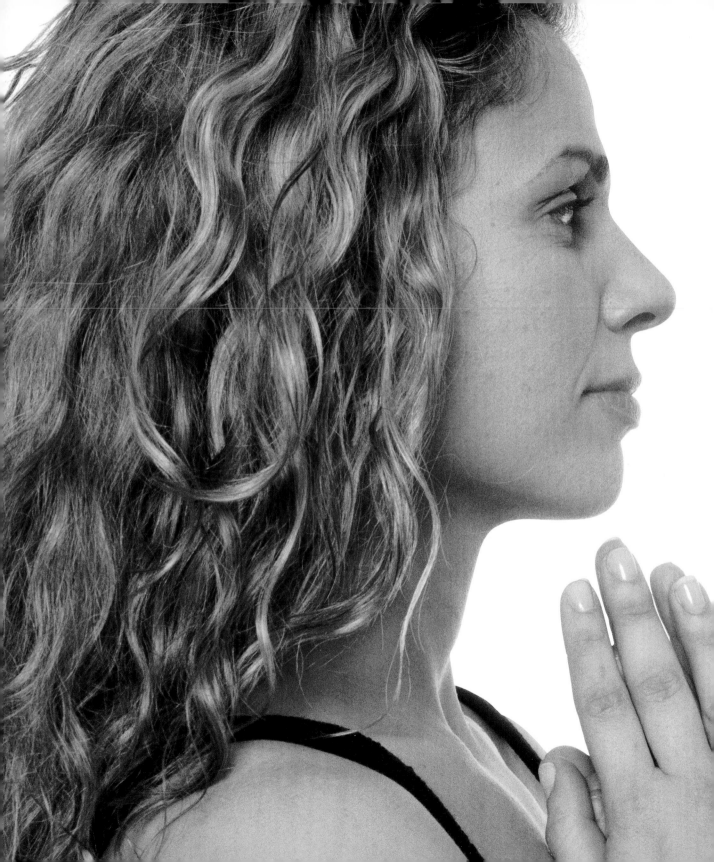

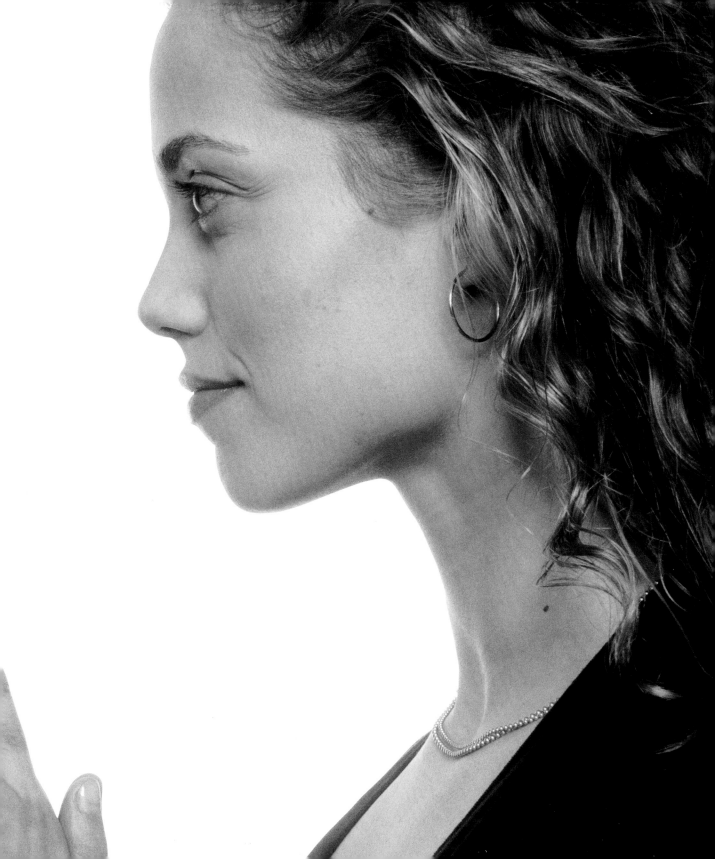

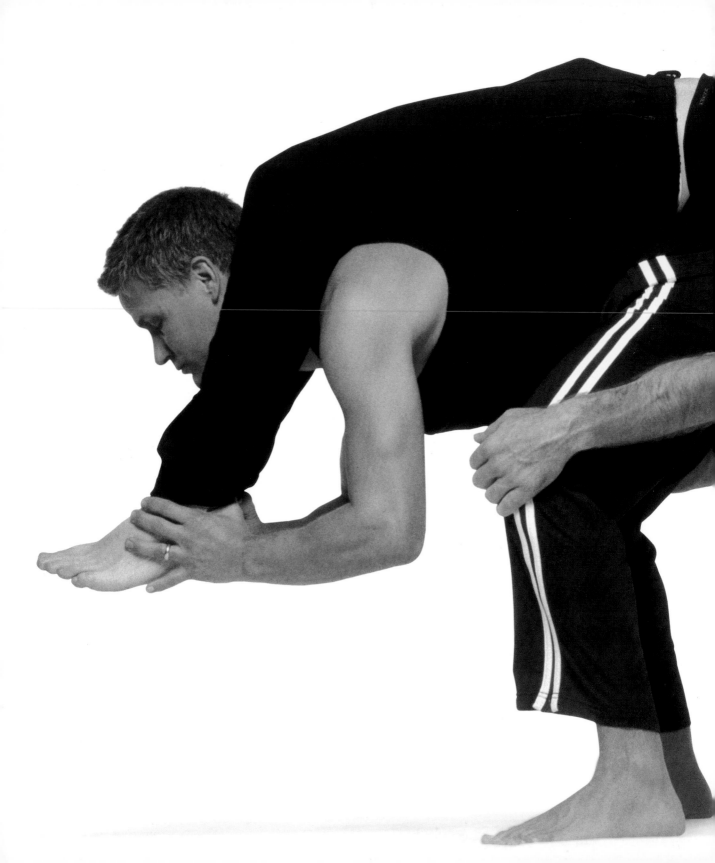

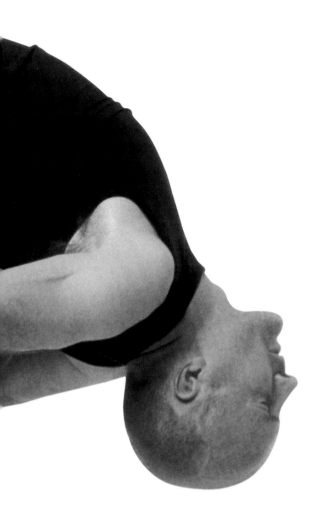

SPINAL ALIGNMENT VARIATION

STEPHEN & DEVARSHI

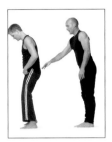

STEP 1 Stephen and Devarshi discuss how to adjust their spacing in order to best support each other.

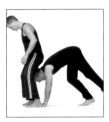

STEP 2 Stephen places his hands behind Devarshi's feet in preparation for a handstand. Devarshi bends his knees to prepare himself to assist.

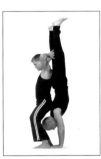

STEP 3 Stephen kicks into a handstand. Devarshi finds his legs.

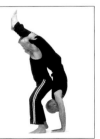

STEP 4 Holding on to Stephen's shins, Devarshi tucks his shoulders into the backs of Stephen's knees and starts to bend forward.

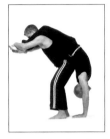

STEP 5 Bending Stephen's knees over his shoulders, Devarshi hooks his arms over Stephen's ankles to pull him forward while simultaneously arching his back.

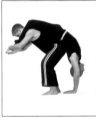

STEP 6 Devarshi continues to fold forward, pulling Stephen into a deep backbend.

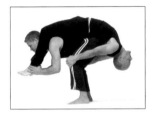

STEP 7 Stephen hangs off Devarshi's back in a deep, heart-opening stretch.

STEP 8 Devarshi squats down, placing his hands on the ground to stabilize himself and to lower Stephen's feet toward the ground. When Stephen is ready to dismount, he places his feet down and stands up.

133

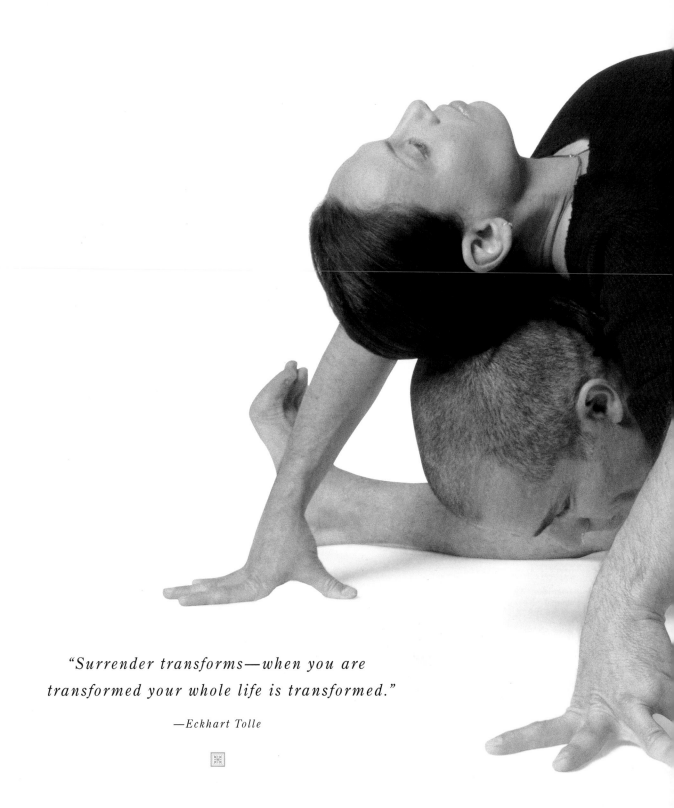

"*Surrender transforms—when you are*
transformed your whole life is transformed."

—*Eckhart Tolle*

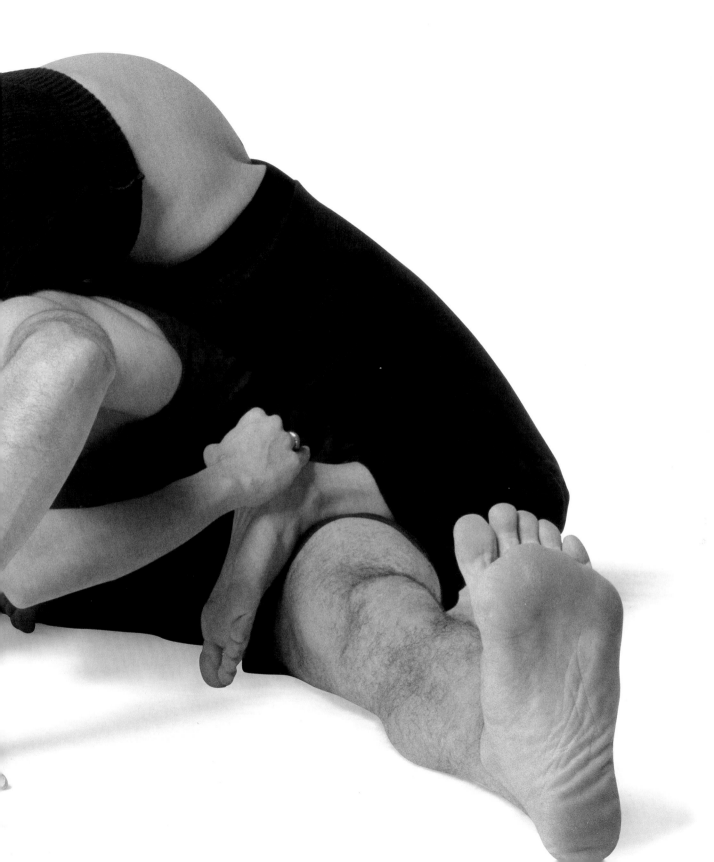

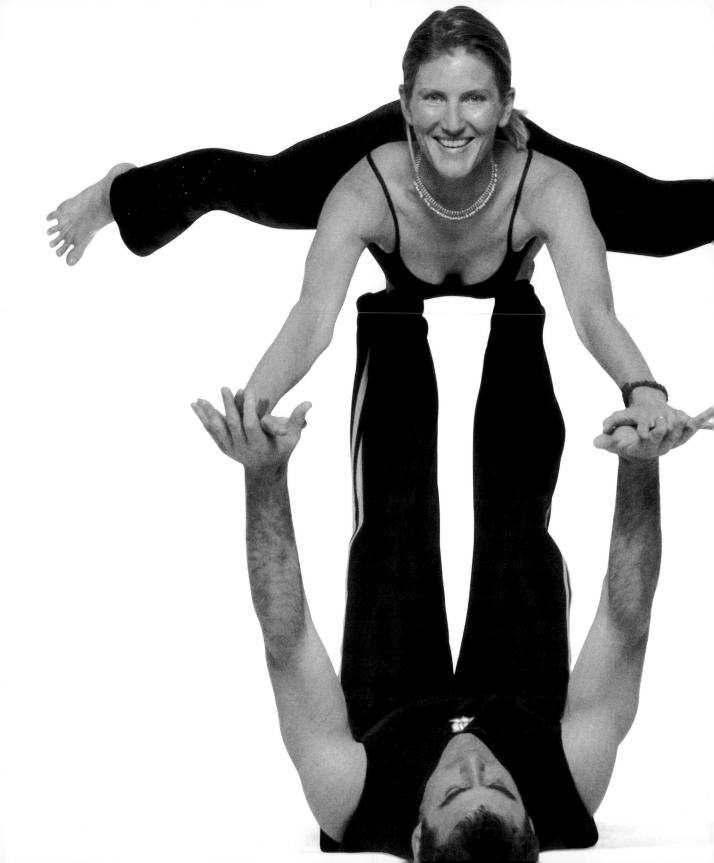

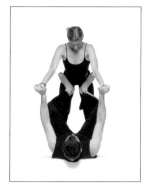

FLYING SPLIT
SHIVA & TIM

STEP 1 Shiva places Tim's feet along her outer hip/thigh creases and leans forward. Tim takes her hands to support her as he bends his knees to take her weight over his center.

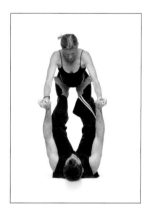

STEP 2 Maintaining eye contact, Tim presses his legs straight, lifting Shiva off the ground, keeping his hands directly above his shoulders.

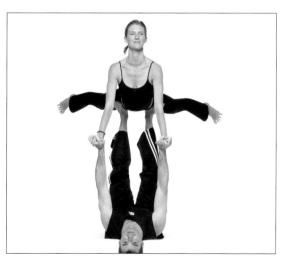

STEP 3 Shiva extends her legs wide as she lifts her chest and her gaze. Fully supported by Tim, she flies.

UNION

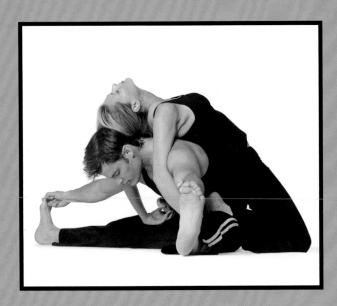

Qualities:

SURRENDER
SERVICE
FREEDOM

Gift:

GRACE

Challenge:

EGO

To achieve true union in a relationship is a remarkable thing. You'll know it when you find it. No one is leading; no one is following. The dance unfolds miraculously, as if orchestrated by a single being. Two become one, and their combined field expands into something far beyond the sum of its parts. It is for these moments that we live and for this ecstasy that we risk the vulnerability of falling in love.

Even though most of us long for this union, we also fear it. We may think it means we have to give up ourselves and get helplessly lost in the other. But it's really just the opposite, for the transcendent state of union brings us closer to the place in which we really find ourselves. To find a beloved is a divine blessing indeed.

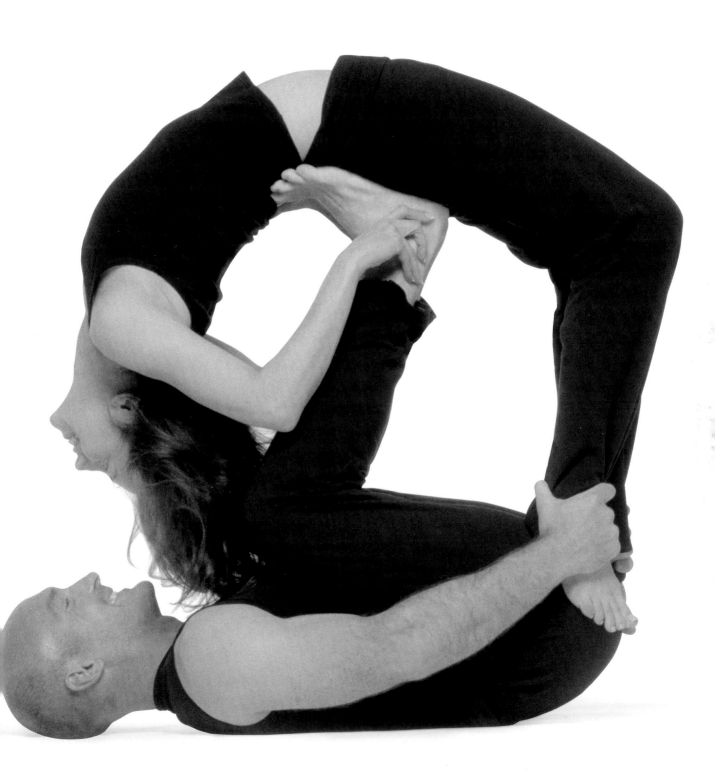

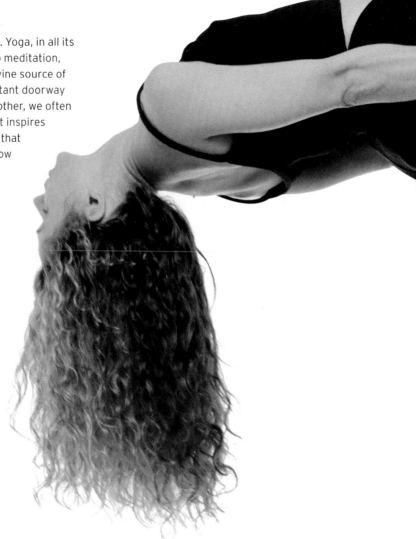

The true meaning of the word *yoga* is union. Yoga, in all its various practices, from asanas to pranayama to meditation, is designed to reunite the individual with the divine source of unified consciousness. Relationship is an important doorway to this experience, for in ecstatic union with another, we often get our first taste of transcendence, a taste that inspires us to enter the deeper mystery of unity with all that is. Relationship can show us what it's like, to know what it is we are seeking.

Transcendence, long held as an ideal in many spiritual traditions, has seldom been applied to relationship, yet there is no greater training ground for transcending the ego and dissolving your boundaries than the infinite dance of relating to another person. Through repeated practice with your partner, through alignment of your bodies, emotions, commitments, love, truth, and visions, you eventually direct your energies into a single pool of divine consciousness, which bathes both of you in bliss.

It is the mind that creates the illusion of separation and the ego that maintains it. To find unity, we must get out of our heads, release the intellect, and enter a state of being. We must overcome the exaggerated importance of the self and enter the divine mystery of spiritual surrender. To achieve this, surrender your preconceived notions, your needs, your ego, your control to serve the transcendent relationship. This is not an abandonment of yourself, but an ecstatic offering of gifts from the individual soul to the universal spirit.

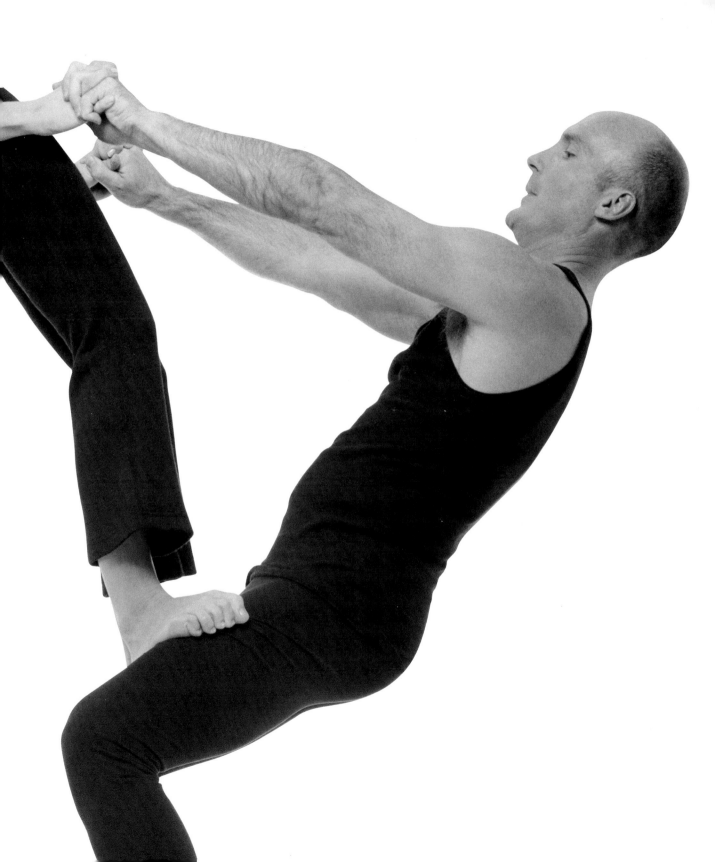

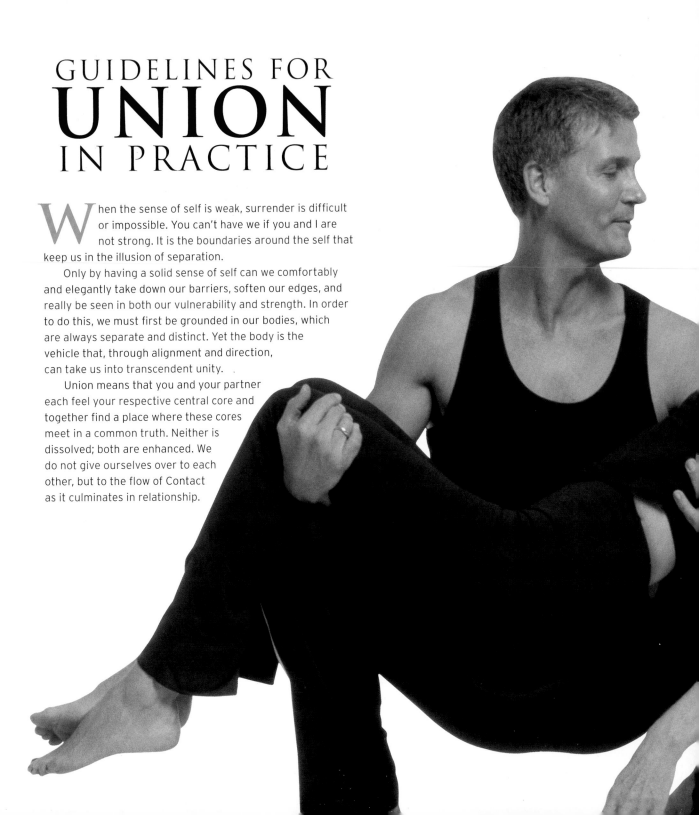

GUIDELINES FOR
UNION
IN PRACTICE

When the sense of self is weak, surrender is difficult or impossible. You can't have we if you and I are not strong. It is the boundaries around the self that keep us in the illusion of separation.

Only by having a solid sense of self can we comfortably and elegantly take down our barriers, soften our edges, and really be seen in both our vulnerability and strength. In order to do this, we must first be grounded in our bodies, which are always separate and distinct. Yet the body is the vehicle that, through alignment and direction, can take us into transcendent unity.

Union means that you and your partner each feel your respective central core and together find a place where these cores meet in a common truth. Neither is dissolved; both are enhanced. We do not give ourselves over to each other, but to the flow of Contact as it culminates in relationship.

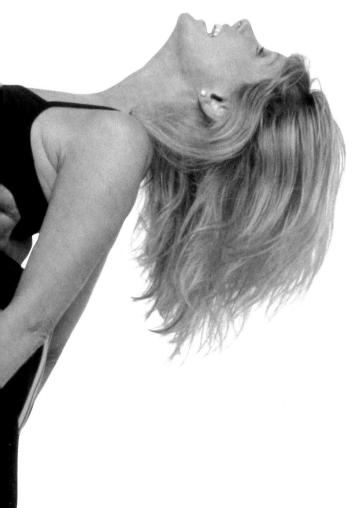

1. **MAKE A STRONG FOUNDATION IN YOUR LEGS,** so that the current is flowing up from the earth, in order to overcome the fear of losing yourself. You must really know how to show up in your practice, be present in your body, and know who you are in relation to your partner. This forms the foundation of trust.

2. **OPEN YOUR BODY TO THE FLOW OF PLEASURE** and passion that begins once trust is established. As the two rivers of consciousness flow toward each other, they begin to merge, sometimes slowly like a great river and sometimes rapidly like white water. Surrender your resistance and harvest the gift of joy. This will enliven your energy to move forward.

3. **AS YOUR RIVERS CRASH INTO EACH OTHER, GUIDE THEM WILLFULLY.** Your commitment firms the banks of these streams to contain the energies you are building. Train your bodies to flow together through repeated practice, through determination, through showing up.

4. **OPEN YOUR HEART.** Enter a state of being, not doing. Breathe together, circulating the breath between you. Soften your body and let your attention explore all the places where you make contact in a pose. Feel how precious and fulfilling that can be. Let each pose be an embrace. Opening up to love expands the stream further by dissolving boundaries and creating the desire to unite.

5. **COMMUNICATE YOUR TRUTHS.** Bring your inner feelings out and find the places where they connect with your partner. Use words to direct the flow, to enhance the contact. Build rapport.

6. **HOLD YOUR VISION.** Find the brightness and beauty in the pose. See the radiance in your partner and find the ways to bring that radiance forward. Use your vision to focus the energy along a shining path from present to future.

7. **SURRENDER TO UNION.** When all of these Points are aligned, expand into the moment and let go. Know that you are sharing this moment as one. Open to the grace of the divine union of Shiva and Shakti in their eternal embrace.

SURRENDER
CATHERINE & CASPER

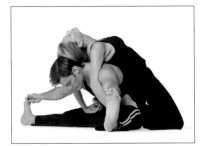

STEP 1 Casper moves into open-leg forward fold, while Catherine squats and then lies over his back, aligning spines.

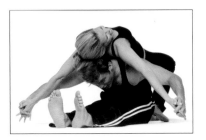

STEP 2 Casper grabs Catherine's hands as she arches over his back, and gently pulls.

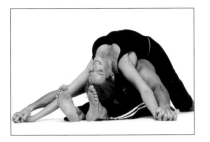

STEP 3 With arms wide and fingers entwined, they breathe, surrender, and relax.

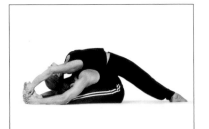

STEP 4 When in Contact, they extend further. Catherine holds Casper's flexed feet and straightens her legs. Casper grabs his own feet and pulls himself deeper into the forward fold.

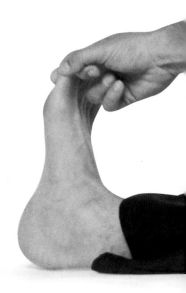

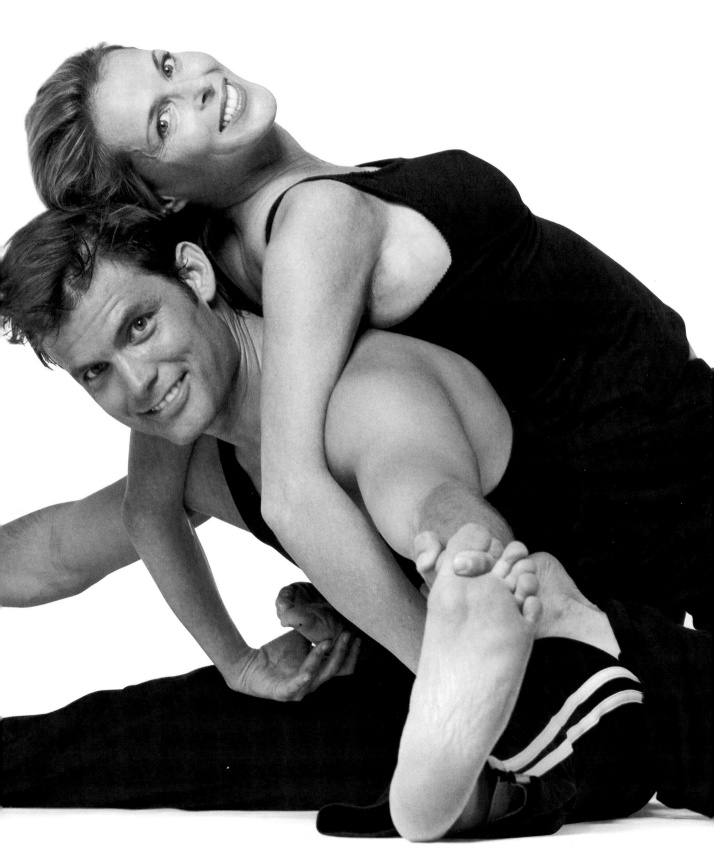

CONTACT
HIGH

Relationship is the spiritual frontier clamoring for attention at this time in our world. While personal spiritual practice is important, even essential, it is not enough to become enlightened alone; we must bring our spiritual growth into relationship with each other, and into our social environment as a whole. The times that are upon us in the world today are desperately calling us to awaken the heart. To open the heart is to relate, and to relate is to embark upon the spiritual challenges of relationship.

Relationship requires contact. Whether between the United States and another country, between races, genders, or belief systems, or just between friends and lovers, contact and connectedness weave the fabric of understanding, harmony, and peace. Without contact, alienation brews, disharmony arises, and enmity occurs.

No one truly lives a solitary life. We embark on relationships in every aspect of our lives—with our coworkers, our neighbors, our family, friends, and partners. Yet conscious relationship is a relatively new invention, something we are just learning about in our culture.

As the world rapidly changes on every level of existence, it is essential to develop new forms for relationships and new ways of relating. In order to do this, we need effective tools for experiencing the spiritual ecstasy that relationship can provide. It is time to take the aspects of solitary spiritual practice and bring them into relationship and into community.

Contact Yoga is an evolutionary step along that path, leading to a discovery of the Beloved in yourself, your partner, and in the divine aspect of life around you. The divine Beloved is always there. Our challenge is to make contact with it, to touch it and taste it, to feel it and see it, to know it and grow with it. To make contact with the Beloved is to feel indescribable joy at simply being alive. To share that aliveness with another is to share a spiritual nectar that brings strength, clarity, and profound peace, opening a gateway that renews what has been lost and opens frontiers not yet discovered.

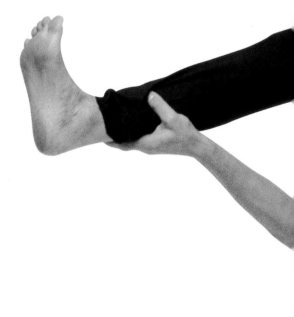

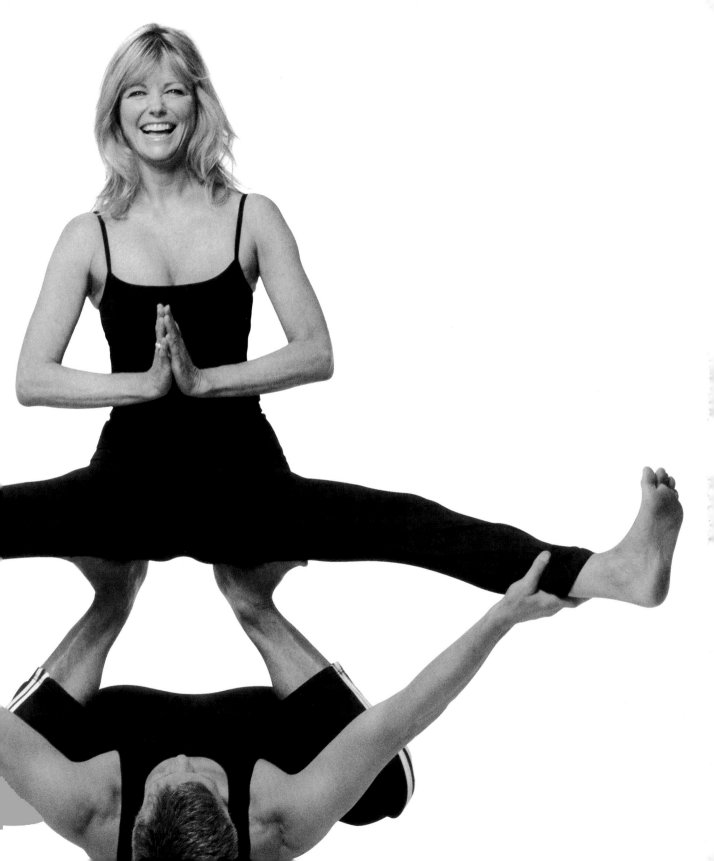

RESTING TORSO OPENER
ANGELA & VICTOR

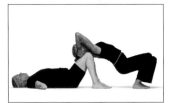

STEP 1 Angela interlaces her fingers behind her neck. She places the curve of her neck on Victor's knees and rests her head on his thighs.

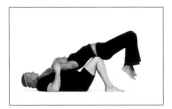

STEP 4 Angela interlaces her fingers behind Victor's neck; he assists her in lifting her legs by supporting her sacrum and pulling her arms into him.

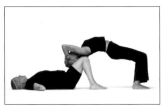

STEP 2 Pressing into her feet, Angela lifts her hips up and starts to slide her back along Victor's knees. He keeps his legs steady.

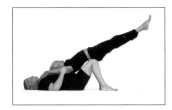

STEP 5 Victor lowers his head, continuing to support Angela as she straightens her legs.

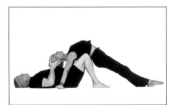

STEP 3 Victor lengthens and massages Angela's neck as she straightens her legs, opening her chest.

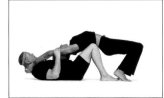

STEP 6 Angela bends her knees and lowers her feet to the ground. She rests, supported by Victor, and stretches her torso open even further from head to hip.

"Take time out to have time in."

—*Tara Guber*

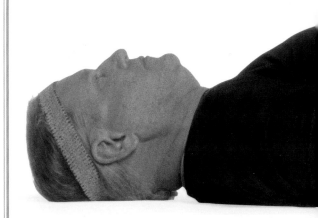

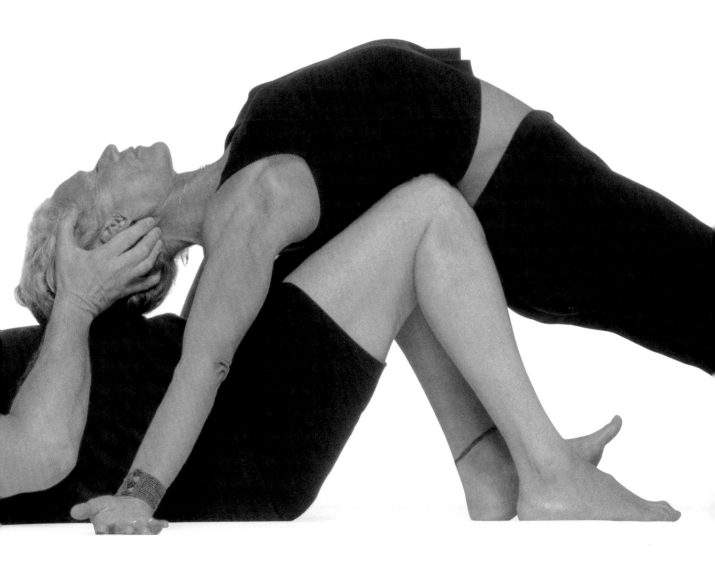

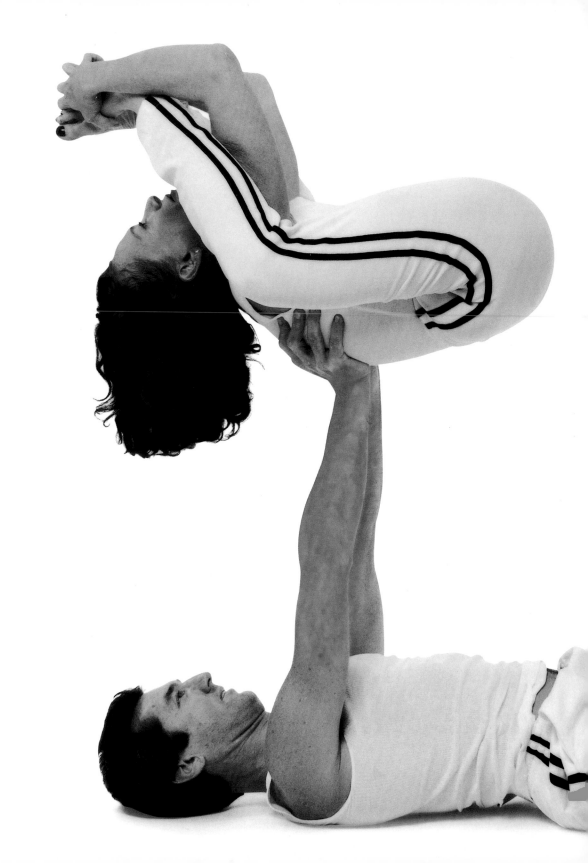

"This moment is as it should be:
Intention has infinite
organizing power."

—*Deepak Chopra*

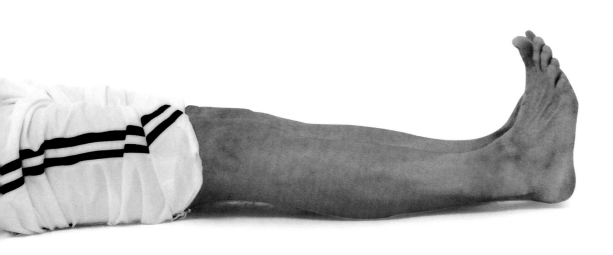

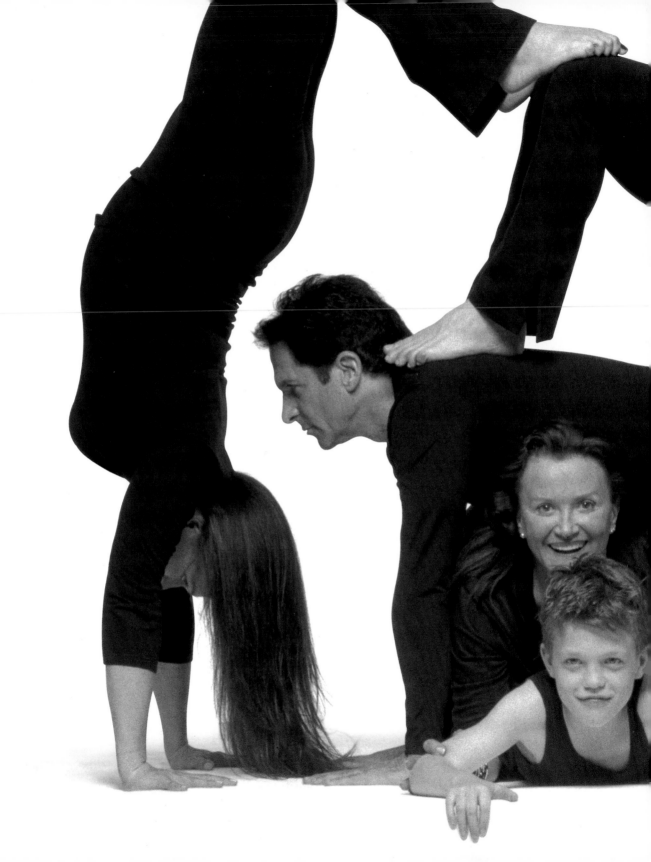

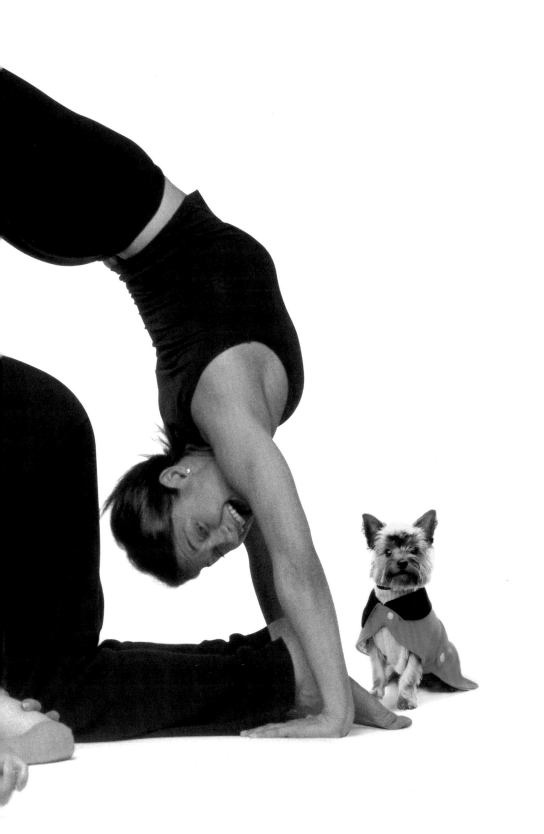

STANDING LOTUS

ANA & SHIVA

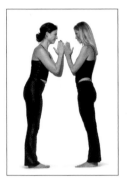

STEP 1 Ana and Shiva greet and connect. They bow and breathe together, linking body, mind, energy, and intention.

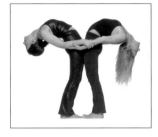

STEP 4 Continuing to stretch and pull simultaneously, they extend into full standing backbends as they slowly straighten their arms.

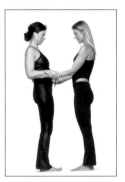

STEP 2 They clasp forearms and move their feet a little closer together.

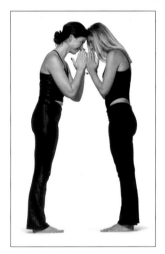

STEP 5 Ana and Shiva slowly come out of standing lotus but stay in the posture, ending more deeply connected than when they began.

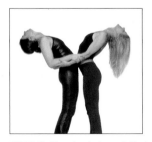

STEP 3 They begin to arch their backs and simultaneously pull in to support each other.

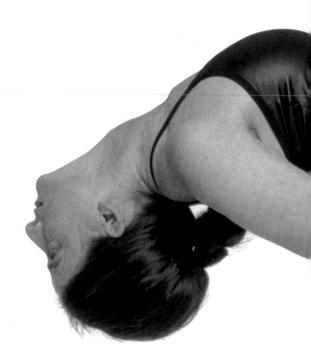

"Exploring the mysterious edge where two people connect physically, emotionally, and spiritually."

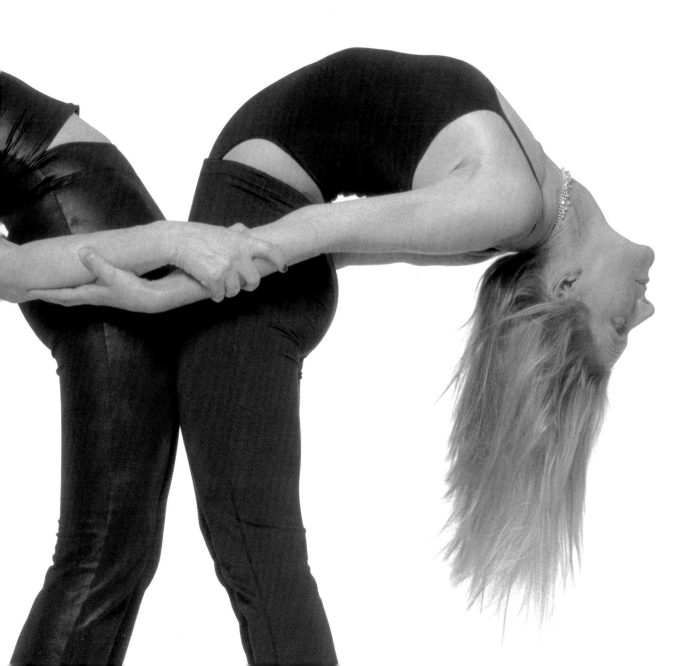

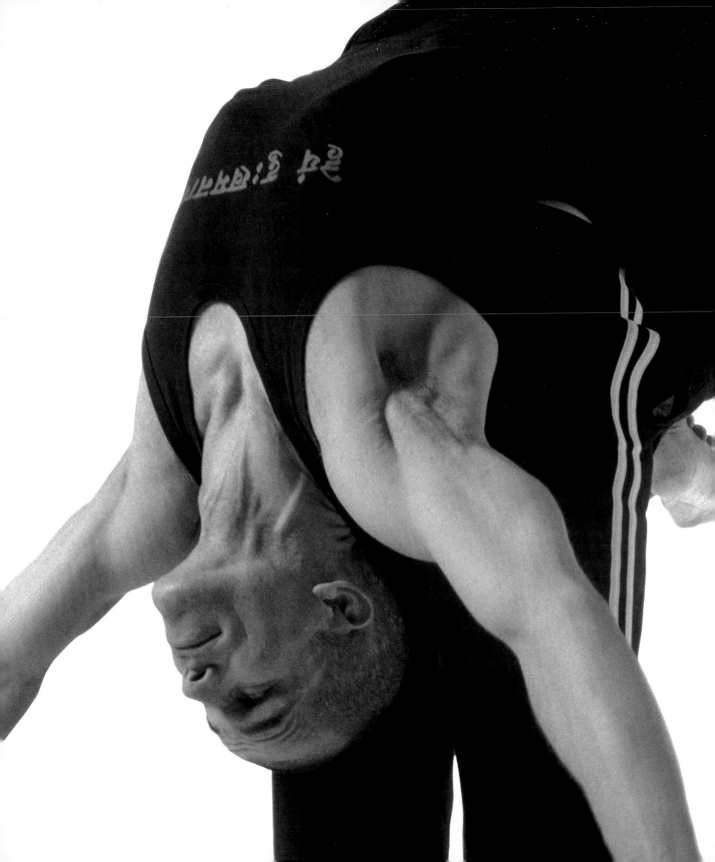

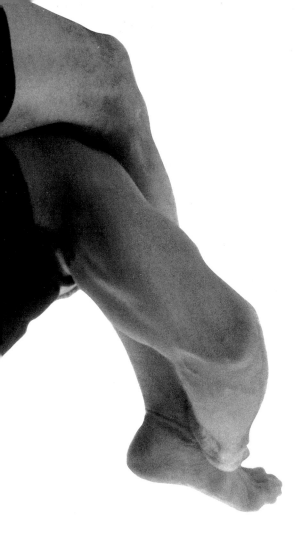

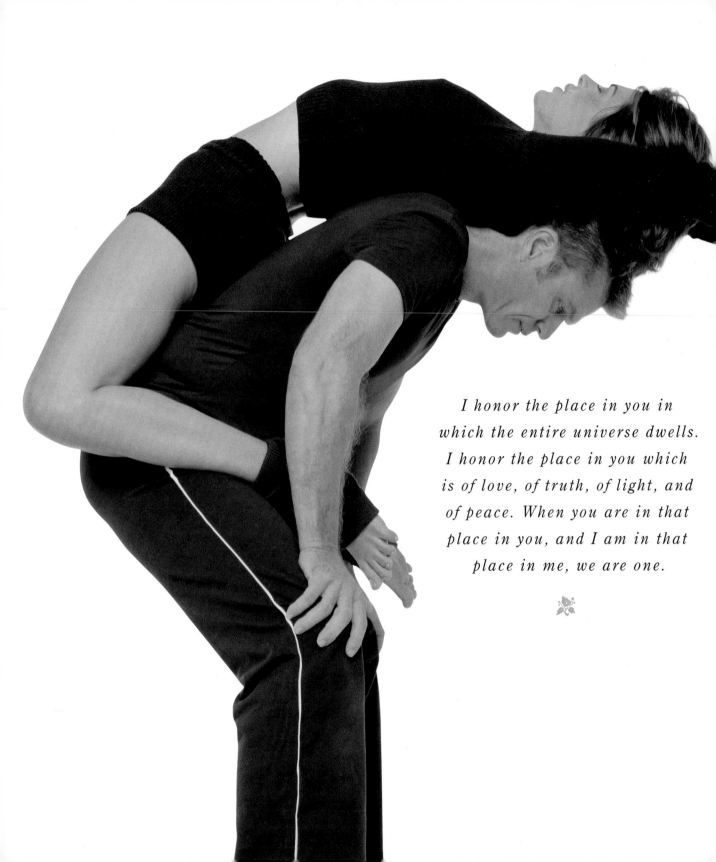

I honor the place in you in which the entire universe dwells. I honor the place in you which is of love, of truth, of light, and of peace. When you are in that place in you, and I am in that place in me, we are one.

THE JOURNEY CONTINUES

Since its first publication, my exploration of relationship through yoga has evolved and expanded, in a large part due to the many people who are now experiencing Contact with the book you hold as their guide. The response to and impact of the work is very heartening, and I'm inspired to hear so many stories of the emotional and energetic breakthroughs and transformations that Contact Yoga has ignited in so many yogis.

But most interesting to me are the comments I hear from non-yogis who are deeply touched by the book's philosophy and are inspired to explore a yoga practice. The Seven Points of Contact inspire the postures in these pages but are not defined by them. As they help two people become one in relationship, so can they help you achieve harmony within yourself.

The truth is, everyone wants Relationship but few want to actually work on it. We tend to feel relationship is only expressed by feelings and emotions but it is actually the expression of a harmony between our mind, heart, and spirit. In yoga, these elements are specifically addressed and brought into balance, making yoga the ideal practice to help you realize the fulfillment, joy, and peace that awaits you in your bond with another.

So here's my advice: bring to the relationship what you desire for yourself in relationship—seek to embody the Seven Points of Contact so you may share that experience with another. The more trusting you choose to be in this process, the more you will manifest the profound gifts of the Seven Points in your relationship.

My journey in Contact and Relationship continues to illuminate my practice and my life; I wish you many discoveries and revelations as you follow your own path to sacred Union.

With love and light,
Tara

THE CONTACT YOGIS

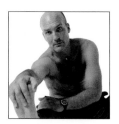

STEPHEN BARTON has been practicing yoga for over fifteen years. He lives in Los Angeles, where he works as a writer and fitness trainer.

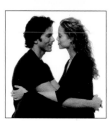

ELIZABETH BERKLEY found success early, landing the role of Jessie on the classic sitcom *Saved By the Bell*. In 1994, she made her big-screen debut as a dancer in *Showgirls*. Her film credits span major Hollywood releases like *The First Wives Club* and *The Curse of the Jade Scorpion* and indie favorites such as *Roger Dodger* and *Moving Malcolm*. She's also appeared on the London stage in *Lenny* and off-Broadway in *Hurlyburly*. **GREG LAUREN**, her husband, is a New York- and Los Angeles–based artist. He has become an emerging talent in the art world with numerous solo exhibitions in the last ten years. Lauren counts such famous names as Ben Stiller, Demi Moore, and Renée Zellweger among his collectors.

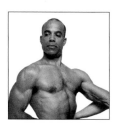

JONATHAN BOWRA studied with Korean Zen Master Seung Sahn for twenty-four years, fourteen of which were spent living in Zen centers doing intensive meditation training. He spent four years as a Buddhist monk. He brings his extensive meditation experience to his practice of yoga, teaching through storytelling, chanting meditation, sitting meditation, and bowing meditation, as well as asanas. Bowra co-teaches Forrest Yoga® with Ana Forrest both nationally and internationally.

SEANE CORN is a renowned yoga instructor at Sacred Movement in Santa Monica, California, and a familiar face in the yoga community: she has been featured in many national commercials, magazines, and DVDs. Her

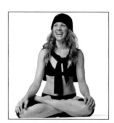

classes integrate vigorous vinyasa flow with alignment, focus, visualization, meditation, and prayer. Corn has studied with healers and spiritual therapists in a variety of disciplines, including Barbara Soloman, Mona Miller, Carolyn Myss, and Anodea Judith. As the National Yoga Ambassador for YouthAIDS, Corn has helped bring awareness to the HIV/AIDS crisis through the "Off the Mat, Into the World" campaign.

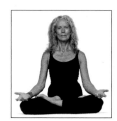

ANGELA FARMER has taught yoga internationally for over four decades. She studied with B.K.S. Iyengar for ten years, making several trips to India, but later developed her own more fluid, personal approach to Hatha Yoga, which fosters dialogue between the body and inner self. Leading workshops and classes around the world with her partner, Victor van Kooten, Farmer has produced two videos, *The Feminine Unfolding* and *A Flow Class with Angela*.

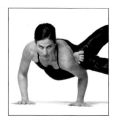

ANA FORREST is the founder of Forrest Yoga®, a Santa Monica-based yoga studio that is home to her uniquely developed method of practice. Born with leg and torso deformities, Forrest's experience of yoga is deeply influenced by her focus on emotional and physical healing. Forrest Yoga® has its roots in many yoga styles and healing modalities, including Native American medicine and ceremony. Forrest is a well-known contributing expert to *Yoga Journal* and other national wellness publications. She teaches internationally at yoga conferences, workshops, and teacher-training sessions.

SHARON GANNON, a renowned teacher around the globe, created the Jivamukti Yoga Method

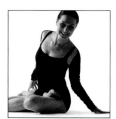

along with David Life in 1984. Jivamukti incorporates vigorous Hatha Yoga classes with the study of ancient texts like the Yoga Sutras of Patanjali and the Upanishads. The seven Jivamukti Yoga centers around the world hold regular meditation sessions and a wide range of workshops, in addition to Sanskrit classes taught and chanted in their traditional forms. Gannon brings a rare blend of scholarly study, artistic pursuit, and highly disciplined asana and meditation practice to her offerings as a teacher. The author of *Cats and Dogs Are People Too*, *Jivamukti Yoga*, and *The Art of Yoga*, Gannon has many high-profile students, including Sting, Russell Simmons, Donna Karan, and Geshe Michael Roach.

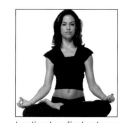

JENNIFER GRANT, actress and daughter of Cary Grant and Dyan Cannon, graduated from Stanford with a degree in history and political science in 1987. She moved into acting in 1993, landing her first role on *Beverly Hills, 90210* and appearing on a variety of television shows, including *Ellen* and *CSI*. She's taught yoga to public school kids from grades six to eleven in Manhattan.

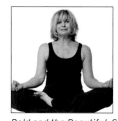

LINDA GRAY, Emmy-nominated actress, is best known for her role as Sue Ellen on the hit television series *Dallas* and has enjoyed a guest-starring role on the popular daytime drama *The Bold and the Beautiful*. Gray made her stage debut alongside Larry Hagman in *Love Letters* and also starred in the London West End's production of *The Graduate*. An Ambassador of Goodwill for the United Nations, Gray has her own production company with several projects in development.

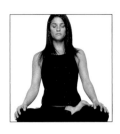

ELIZABETH GUBER, daughter of Tara Guber, has an MA in Clinical Psychology and is a research psychologist on the ADHD Genetic Study at UCLA. She practices psychology at the Maple Counseling Center in Beverly Hills and co-leads anger-management groups for teenagers at Beverly Hills High School.

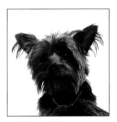

GUS YORK GUBER I is a rare breed of Yorkshire Terrier born and raised in the City of Angels. Practically all nine pounds of Gus are a combination of his uniquely disproportionate ear size and his enormous personality. Gus developed an affinity for yoga following a near-death experience with a coyote when he was only a baby Yorkie. He attributes his escape from the coyote's jowls to his innate canine genetics, which allowed him to propel himself to safety by adjusting himself in an intense downward dog. After such a victory, Gus stayed true to yoga and every morning, he downward dogs now. It has made his life all the richer, and he is honored to be part of the yoga community!

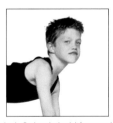

JAXON GUBER, son of Tara Guber, enthusiastically participated in the making of this book as a twelve-year-old. A regular practitioner of yoga and meditation with his mom and dad, Guber's hobbies past and present include playing guitar, basketball, baseball, and soccer. He continues to enjoy spending family time with his parents and siblings.

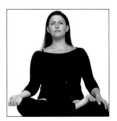

JODI GUBER, daughter of Tara Guber, is the driving force behind the creation of Beyond, a multi-faceted lifestyle, clothing, and jewelry company made up of the brands Beyond Yoga and Beyond Malas. She teaches Anusara-inspired vinyasa flow, a style of Hatha Yoga that works both the inner and outer body, encouraging an opening of the heart while strongly working with the principles of alignment. Her students come to her for the inner healing she offers through her words, touch, and spirit.

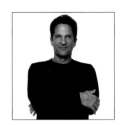

PETER GUBER, husband of Tara Guber, is the chairman and CEO of the Mandalay Entertainment Group, which specializes in motion pictures, television, sports entertainment, and new media. Over the course of his illustrious thirty-five-year career, Guber's films have earned more than $3 billion worldwide and more than fifty Academy Award nominations, including a Best Picture Oscar win for *Rain Man*. He is a sought-after speaker and appeared Sunday mornings as the cohost of the critically acclaimed AMC's *Sunday Morning Shootout*, a show is based on his best-selling book. Guber is a full professor at the UCLA School of Theater, Film, and Television, and has been a member of the faculty for over three decades.

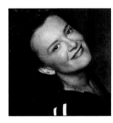

TARA GUBER, a teacher, producer, and philanthropist, is the founder and president of the nationally recognized yoga-in-schools program Yoga Ed. She is a founding board member of the Accelerated School, the internationally recognized charter public school in South Central Los Angeles, named "Elementary School of the Year" in 2001 by *Time* magazine. Guber has studied yoga for over thirty-five years and Contact Yoga for twenty years. She's taught classes across the United States and Canada. Contact Yoga has been featured in numerous publications, including *Yoga Journal, Women's Wear Daily, Self, Time, InStyle, Rolling Stone*, and *Healing Retreats and Spas*. Guber makes her home with her family in Los Angeles, California.

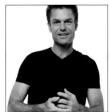

HARRY HAMLIN, *People*'s Sexiest Man Alive in 1987, studied acting at San Francisco's American Conservatory Theatre. He's appeared in numerous films and television shows. Hamlin is best known for his role as attorney Michael Kuzak on the television drama *L.A. Law*. and appeared regularly on TV's *Veronica Mars*. He and his wife, Lisa Rinna, live in Los Angeles with their two daughters.

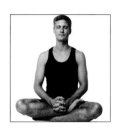

DEVARSHI/STEVEN HARTMAN, RYT, is the Director of Professional Trainings and Yoga Teacher Trainer at the Kripalu center based in Lenox, Massachusetts. A yoga student and teacher for over twenty-five years, Devarshi is the creator of the best-selling audio series *The Essence of the Bhagavad Gita*. He leads workshops and retreats and maintains a private practice in Chicago, where he is a bodyworker, teacher, and practitioner of the healing arts.

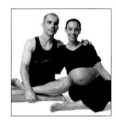

NAIME JEZZENY and **SUE ELKIND** are both nationally renowned senior certified Anusara Yoga teachers who are celebrated for their inspiring, accessible, and detailed teaching method. Jezzeny and Elkind relocated from Los Angeles to Bucks County, Pennsylvania, with their two boys, Luca and Milo. They teach classes, workshops, and trainings at Yogaphoria™, in their hometown of New Hope, Pennsylvania, as well as across the nation.

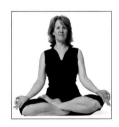

ANODEA JUDITH discovered yoga in 1975 when she first began writing about chakras, culminating in her classic book, *Wheels of Life: A User's Guide to the Chakra System* (with over two hundred fifty thousand copies in print). She has become a leading authority on the subject with numerous books and products, including the groundbreaking psychology text *Eastern Body, Western Mind* and the award-winning video *The Illuminated Chakras*. She is a widely acclaimed workshop leader, somatic therapist, and yoga teacher, with a master's in Clinical Psychology and a PhD in Mind-Body Healing. Her newest book is entitled *Waking the Global Heart*.

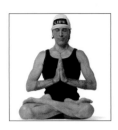

DAVID LIFE has taught yoga for more than twenty years throughout the United States and around the world. His interest in yoga is supported by his artistic, literary, and metaphysical studies. Life is a certified Advanced Level II practitioner of the Ashtanga system of Shri K. Pattabhi Jois of Mysore, India. He studied yoga with many gurus, including Shri Brahmananda Saraswati, Shri Swami Nirmalananda, and Shri K. Pattabhi Jois. He spent several years as a *sannyas* (renunciate) of a lineage of yogic monks in India and has received Kalachakra and Bodhisattva initiation from His Holiness the 14th Dalai Lama. Together with Sharon Gannon, he has created the Jivamukti Yoga Method, which focuses on teaching and practicing yoga as a means to enlightenment.

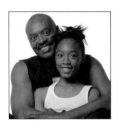

REGGIE MAEWEATHER served in the Los Angeles Police Department for thirty years. He served as captain for many of those years, before retiring in August 2004. As the senior commanding officer in Newton Area, Maeweather was responsible for one of the most violent and crime-ridden areas of the city. His prime initiative was to reduce crime by building strong relationships in the residential, business, and political communities throughout the city. As a divorced father of two, Maeweather lovingly spent the majority of his subsequent years raising his sixteen-year-old daughter, Adrienne. He lives in Phillips Ranch, California.

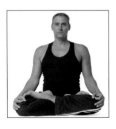

VINNIE MARINO is a high-profile vinyasa flow teacher in Los Angeles who began practicing yoga as a teenager in New York. He took his first teacher training at the White Lotus Foundation in Santa Barbara. In 1997, he completed the Yoga Works Teacher Training and has since completed his second YW Teacher Training and the Advanced Teacher Training Program. He also appeared as a featured model in the health section of the *Los Angeles Times*. Marino teaches a strong, physically challenging practice set to great music with a playful attitude.

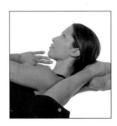

RAINBEAU MARS is the creator, writer, and coproducer of the *Yoga for Beauty* series, *Dusk and Dawn*, prenatal best seller *ZenMama*, and the four-part, nationally acclaimed *Sacred Yoga* series: *Pure Power, Sweat, Tranquility*, and *Yoga for Beginners*. Mars has been on the covers of *Body and Soul, Yoga Journal, Elephant*, and *New Living*, and has appeared in publications such as *Shape, Fitness, YogiTimes*, and *Delicious*. As the daughter of renowned author/herbalist Brigitte Mars, she was taught the power of self-healing at an early age; her work and her life are dedicated to helping her clients, students, and friends learn the benefits of this lifestyle.

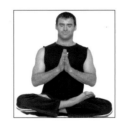

TED MCDONALD is a yoga teacher, endurance athlete, and freelance writer. He founded Adventure Yoga Retreats, a company that assists yoga teachers in organizing, marketing, and administrating their yoga retreats worldwide. Educated in both Iyengar and Ashtanga, he teaches a vinyasa flow class with upbeat music, creating a fun and safe environment for his students. The growth of his yoga business is connected to McDonald's entrepreneurial skills as well as his ability to successfully tailor his teaching and retreats to a diverse audience, including endurance athletes, business professionals, yoga teachers, and beginning students.

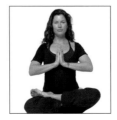

CARRÉ OTIS began modeling at the age of fifteen, has been photographed by the world's most famous photographers, and has graced the covers of dozens of magazines, including *Elle, Vogue*, and *Harper's Bazaar*. Introduced to yoga at seventeen, Otis found herself stepping onto the path of Tibetan Buddhism. Today, she is recognized as an expert on health, recovery, and self-discovery. An in-demand public speaker, she frequently travels the country to address middle school, high school, and college audiences. Otis is also a spokesperson for the National Eating Disorders Association.

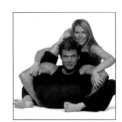

CATHERINE OXENBERG rose to fame on the hit show *Dynasty*, and since then has appeared in more than twenty films. **CASPER VAN DIEN** starred in *Starship Troopers, Tarzan*, and *Sleepy Hollow*. Oxenberg and Van Dien are partners in a production company that focuses on ways to uplift humanity through media. They also survived a thirteen-episode reality show for Lifetime TV called *I Married a Princess*. The two are devoted philanthropists and the ecstatic parents of five children.

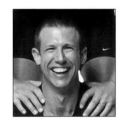

JULES PAXTON holds a master of science in Foreign Service from Georgetown University and studied law at Columbia University. Inspired by his experiences in competitive bodybuilding, he embraced yoga and other spiritual practices as a wellspring for tapping into his own human potential. His innovative approach to alignment has made him a highly sought-after empowerment practitioner. He is also an author who explores the topic of the human body and its infinite potential.

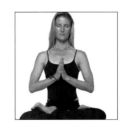

SHIVA REA is a global yogini exploring the roots and branches of yoga as a universal path. She teaches vinyasa flow worldwide. Rea's studies in the Krishnamacharya lineage, Tantra, ayurveda, yogic art, and somatic movement all inform her approach to living yoga and embodying flow. A regular contributor to *Yoga Journal*, she has led over sixty retreats and pilgrimages in Asia, Africa, and the Caribbean. She is the Creative Yoga Director of Exhale Spa and has produced several popular yoga DVDs. Rea lives with her family in Los Angeles, where she teaches at Sacred Movement and UCLA.

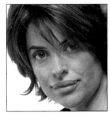

LISA RINNA, an Emmy-nominated actress, has been practicing yoga for over twelve years. Rinna has appeared on *Days of Our Lives*, *Melrose Place*, *Soaptalk*, and *Dancing with the Stars*. She and her husband, Harry Hamlin, live in Los Angeles with their two daughters.

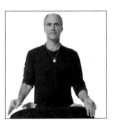

STEVE ROSS has practiced various styles of yoga for more than thirty years and has been an instructor for over twenty of them. He spent four years as a monk in the Vedic tradition, and since then he has sought out some of the most notable masters of our time in India and elsewhere. Ross employs upbeat, inspirational music and a relaxed, easy spirituality to make his classes at MahaYoga some of the most popular in Los Angeles.

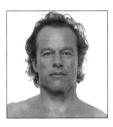

ROD STRYKER has taught Tantra, Hatha, and Yogananda's Kriya Yoga for more than twenty years. In addition to leading trainings and retreats worldwide, Stryker specializes in the art of personalizing yoga and meditation practices for individuals. He is on the advisory board of *Yoga International* as well as *Healing Retreats and Spas* magazines and serves on the board of directors of the Himalayan Institute in Honesdale, Pennsylvania. He's been a consultant to corporations on the benefits of yoga, taught yoga and meditation alongside Deepak Chopra, and developed a video series entitled *Yoga for Longevity*. He has also produced the highly acclaimed guided meditation CD *3 Meditations to Live By*.

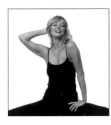

CHERYL TIEGS, best known as the "All-American Model," is also an author, businesswoman, and avid spokesperson for women's health, the environment, and underprivileged children. She continues to model frequently, appears in public for speaking engagements and on television, and has launched a line of skin-care products. A sought-after speaker on the subjects of health, fitness, and living a balanced life, Tiegs also travels regularly to third-world countries as a charitable ambassador on behalf of the United Nations. She lives in Los Angeles, California.

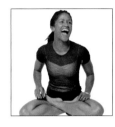

BAHNI TURPIN discovered Hatha Yoga in the '80s, after an exploration into metaphysics, meditation, drama, and dance, when she attended a Jivamukti class taught by David Life. When she moved to Los Angeles, she attended her first "flow"-style class and became hooked on its dance-like rhythm. In 1997, Turpin attended teacher training at Yoga Works in Santa Monica and soon after began teaching at Paramount Studios. Currently, she teaches privately and at Yoga Works.

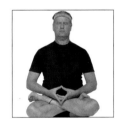

VICTOR VAN KOOTEN began studying yoga at the age of twenty-seven with B.K.S. Iyengar and trained to become a yoga teacher. In 1984, van Kooten joined with Angela Farmer and produced a series of books, *Yoga from the Inside Out*, which illuminates yogic teachings.

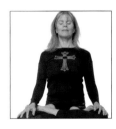

PATRICIA WALDEN is a prominent teacher of classical Iyengar Yoga. Her first instructor was Sufi master Murshid Samuel Lewis, who taught her about the spirituality of dance. Since 1976, she has been a student of B.K.S. Iyengar. She travels annually to Pune, India, to study with him, as well as with his children, Geeta and Prashant Iyengar. Walden, who holds one of few senior advanced Iyengar Yoga teaching certificates in America, is featured in a selection of *Yoga Journal* videos. She has been cited by numerous publications, including *Time* and *Yoga Journal*, for her work with yoga and healing, with the latter naming her "one of twenty-five American yoga originals who are shaping yoga today."

Along with her teaching, Walden is known for her writings, including *The Woman's Book of Yoga and Health* with Linda Sparrowe. She recently closed the B.K.S. Iyengar Yoga Studio in Somerville, Massachusetts, which she cofounded and ran for seventeen years, and she was formerly the president of the B.K.S. Iyengar Yoga Association of Massachusetts. She lives and continues to teach in Boston.

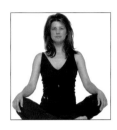

DAPHNE ZUNIGA began her show-business career with a local theater company in Woodstock, Vermont. After studying acting at the American Conservatory Theatre in San Francisco and at UCLA, she gained notice in *The Sure Thing*, *Spaceballs*, and *Last Rites*. In 1992, she joined the cast of the prime-time soap *Melrose Place*, where she played Jo Reynolds, and from 2005-2006 starred in the ABC Family series *Beautiful People*.

ACKNOWLEDGMENTS

When the work speaks to you, you remember all those
who served the work and for whom you are grateful:

My husband, Peter Guber, whose partnership has given me a strong foundation to write a book on relationship, for the freedom he gives me to create, the acceptance he has of my journey, and his unconditional love.

My four children, who are the stars in my life and best friends; Jodi, Elizabeth, Sammy, and Jaxon, all are the most profound blessings in my life.

My mother, Mussie Gellis, who at 100 years was an inspiration to us all.

My Contact Yoga partner, Ken "Tesh" Scott, with whom I learned the meaning of true service and devotion.

My longtime friend and fellow traveler on the path, Norman Seeff, for his fantastic photos and deep commitment to personal growth.

My work partner, Robert Gould, for his service, support, and dedication.

Special thanks to Anodea Judith: a great friend, writer, and yoga partner.

My dear friend Deepak Chopra for his many great insights along the way; Tony Robbins for his passion, wisdom, support, and friendship; the friendships and teachings of Swami Satchidananda, the Dalai Lama, Sharon Salzberg, Catherine Ingram, Caroline Myss, Joseph Michael Levry (Gurunam), Margot Anand, and Romio Shrestha; Catherine Politte, Stephen Barton, Devarshi (Steven Hartman), Kristina Hurrell, Arielle Ford, Ranjana Serle, Seane Corn, Georgina O'Farrill, Lynn Nesbit; Estee Stanley and Christina Ehrlich for styling; Peter Ishkhans and Patrick Jagaille for hair; Lauren Kaye Cohen and Carrie Lynn Orr for makeup; and Beyond Yoga, Carushka, Gaiam, Norma Kamali, and Roots for apparel.

Mandala Publishing, who gave Contact "life" in this book, especially Raoul Goff and Lisa Fitzpatrick. All of my yogini and yogi friends who give of their time to make Contact!

A portion of the proceeds from sales of this book will be donated to Yoga Ed., an organization that brings the benefits of yoga to schools. For more information about Yoga Ed., please visit: www.YogaEd.com.

In the light with love,
Tara

For more information about Contact Yoga, please visit:
www.contactyoga.com.